GET THROUGH

First FRCR:
Questions for the Anatomy Module

Dr Grant Mair – BSc (Hons), MB ChB, MRCS
Specialist Trainee in Radiology: The Royal Infirmary of Edinburgh, UK
Previously, Anatomy Demonstrator: Otago University, Dunedin, New Zealand

Dr Andrew J Baird – MB ChB, MRCS
Specialist Trainee in Radiology: The Royal Infirmary of Edinburgh, UK

Consultant editors
Dr Judith M Anderson – MB ChB, MRCP, MSc, FRCR
Consultant Radiologist: The Royal Infirmary of Edinburgh, UK

Dr Gordon S Findlater – BSc (Hons), PhD
Head of Anatomy: University of Edinburgh, UK

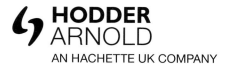

HODDER
ARNOLD
AN HACHETTE UK COMPANY

First published in Great Britain in 2011 by
Hodder Arnold, an imprint of Hodder Eduction, an Hachette UK company,
338 Euston Road, London NW1 3BH

http://www.hoddereducation.com

Hachette UK's policy is to use papers that are natural, renewable and recyclable products and made from wood grown in sustainable forests. The logging and manufacturing processes are expected to conform to the environmental regulations of the country of origin.

Whilst the advice and information in this book are believed to be true and accurate at the date of going to press, neither the author[s] nor the publisher can accept any legal responsibility or liability for any errors or omissions that may be made. In particular (but without limiting the generality of the preceding disclaimer) every effort has been made to check drug dosages; however it is still possible that errors have been missed. Furthermore, dosage schedules are constantly being revised and new side-effects recognized. For these reasons the reader is strongly urged to consult the drug companies' printed instructions before administering any of the drugs recommended in this book.

British Library Cataloguing in Publication Data
A catalogue record for this book is available from the British Library

Library of Congress Cataloging-in-Publication Data
A catalog record for this book is available from the Library of Congress

ISBN-13   978-1-853-15958-9

1 2 3 4 5 6 7 8 9 10

Commissioning Editor: Francesca Naish
Production Controller: Joanna Walker
Cover Designer: Helen Townson
Project management provided by Naughton Project Management

Typeset in 10 pt Minion by Phoenix Photosetting, Chatham, Kent ME4 4TZ
Printed and bound in the UK by CPI Anthony Rowe

What do you think about this book? Or any other Hodder Arnold title?
Please visit our website: www.hodderarnold.com

CONTENTS

Preface   vii

Bibliography   viii

Abbreviations   ix

1 HEAD AND NECK	Questions	1
	Answers	41
2 THORAX	Questions	64
	Answers	94
3 UPPER LIMB	Questions	116
	Answers	136
4 ABDOMEN	Questions	147
	Answers	168
5 PELVIS	Questions	183
	Answers	202
6 LOWER LIMB	Questions	212
	Answers	232
7 MOCK EXAM	Questions	246
	Answers	266

Index   276

This book is dedicated to Suzanne and Mairi,
to thank them for their patience.

PREFACE

Early in 2010 the Royal College of Radiologists re-introduced anatomy as a separate module in the First FRCR examination to be completed in conjunction with the revised physics module which was introduced the previous year. Anatomy is now examined in an electronic image viewing session. Candidates are required to answer a total of 100 questions based on the anatomy identifiable in a series of 20 different radiological images (5 questions per image) sourced from a variety of modalities: namely, radiography, fluoroscopy, ultrasound, CT and MRI (including multi-planar sections). Notably, endoscopic/body cavity ultrasound and nuclear medical images are excluded from this new anatomy syllabus. Further detailed information relating to the examination can be viewed on the Royal College website at www.rcr.ac.uk.

We are both Specialty Trainees in Radiology on the South East Scotland training scheme. When compiling this book we have endeavoured to recreate the question format that candidates are likely to encounter in the anatomy module of the First FRCR examination. Answers and explanations are provided for each question, and while these are not exhaustive, it is hoped that they will clarify the salient anatomical points and form a basis for further reading if required. Unless otherwise stated, our explanations were written with reference to the anatomical textbooks listed in the bibliography. While attempting to cover the curriculum we have also concentrated on subject areas felt to be most important or relevant, in addition to including what could be termed 'exam favourites'. Chapters are divided according to anatomical regions rather than body systems as this is more representative of the imaging that is encountered in everyday practice. As a result, some of the systems (e.g. vascular, neurological and spinal) are covered over two or more chapters.

Dr Judith Anderson is Consultant Radiologist at the Royal Infirmary of Edinburgh and an Educational Supervisor for the South East Scotland radiology training scheme.

Dr Gordon Findlater is Head of the Department of Anatomy at the University of Edinburgh. Both have maintained great enthusiasm for this project in spite of the frequent challenges, problems and deadlines presented to them by the authors. Their guidance and assistance have been essential to the creation of this book and we are indebted to them both.

Finally, we wish you every success in the exam!

Grant Mair
Andrew Baird
Edinburgh

BIBLIOGRAPHY

Abrahams PH, Hutchings RT and Marks SC. *McMinn's Color Atlas of Human Anatomy*, 4th Ed. London: Mosby, 1998

Alty J, Hoey E, Wolstenhulme S and Weston M. *Practical Ultrasound: an Illustrated Guide*. London: RSM Press, 2006

Butler P, Mitchell A and Ellis H. *Applied Radiological Anatomy*. Cambridge: Cambridge University Press, 2007

Hansen JT. *Netter's Anatomy Flash Cards*, 2nd Ed. Philadelphia: Saunders Elsevier, 2007

Marieb EN and Hoehn KH. *Human Anatomy & Physiology*, 7th Ed. San Francisco: Pearson Education, 2007

Moore KL and Agur AMR. *Essential Clinical Anatomy*. Baltimore: Williams & Wilkins, 1996

Raby N, Berman L and de Lacey G. *Accident and Emergency Radiology: A Survival Guide*. Philadelphia: Saunders Elsevier, 2003

Ryan S, McNicholas M and Eustace S. *Anatomy for Diagnostic Imaging*, 2nd Ed. Philadelphia: Saunders Elsevier, 2004

Sinnatamby CS. *Last's Anatomy Regional and Applied*, 10th Ed. Edinburgh: Churchill Livingstone Harcourt, 2001

Standring S. *Gray's Anatomy, The Anatomical Basis of Clinical Practice, Expert Consult – Online and Print*, 40th Ed. Philadelphia: Churchill Livingstone Elsevier, 2008

Weir J, Abrahams PH, Spratt JD and Salkowski LR. *Imaging Atlas of Human Anatomy*, 4th Ed. Philadelphia: Mosby Elsevier, 2010

Weissleder R, Wittenberg J, Harisinghani MG and Chen JW. *Primer of Diagnostic Imaging*, 4th Ed. Philadelphia: Mosby Elsevier, 2007

ABBREVIATIONS

ACJ	Acromioclavicular joint	MLO	Medio-lateral oblique
ACL	Anterior cruciate ligament	mm	Millimetre
AIIS	Anterior inferior iliac spine	MRA	Magnetic resonance angiography
AP	Antero-posterior		
ASIS	Anterior superior iliac spine	MRCP	Magnetic resonance cholangiopancreatography
AV	Atrio-ventricular		
C1–8	Cervical spinal levels (C8 is neural level only)	MRI	Magnetic resonance imaging
CBD	Common bile duct	N1–3	Cancer staging criteria for lymph nodes
CFV	Common femoral vein		
CISS	Constructive interface in steady state (gradient echo MRI sequence)	OM	Occipito-mental
		OPG	Orthopantomogram
		PA	Postero-anterior or pulmonary artery
cm	Centimetre		
CN I–XII	Cranial nerves 1–12	PB	Peroneus brevis
CRL	Crown-rump length	PCL	Posterior cruciate ligament
CSF	Cerebrospinal fluid	PDA	Posterior descending artery
CT	Computed tomography	PL	Peroneus longus
CTPA	CT pulmonary angiogram	PUJ	Pelvi-ureteric junction
CXR	Chest x-ray	PV	Pulmonary veins
DDH	Developmental dysplasia of the hip	RAO	Right anterior oblique
		RCA	Right coronary artery
EDL	Extensor digitorum longus	S1–5	Sacral spinal levels
EHL	Extensor hallucis longus	SA	Sino-atrial
FDL	Flexor digitorum longus	SCM	Sternocleidomastoid
FDP	Flexor digitorum profundus	SI	Sacro-iliac
FDS	Flexor digitorum superficialis	SMA	Superior mesenteric artery
		SMV	Superior mesenteric vein
FHL	Flexor hallucis longus	SVC	Superior vena cava
IAM	Internal auditory meatus	T1–12	Thoracic spinal levels
IMA	Inferior mesenteric artery	T1W/T2W	T1/T2 weighted MRI
IV	Intravenous	TA	Tibialis anterior
IVC	Inferior vena cava	TMJ	Temporomandibular joint
IVU	Intravenous urogram	TP	Tibialis posterior
L1–5	Lumbar spinal levels	True FISP	True fast imaging with steady state precession (MRI sequence)
LAD	Left anterior descending		
LAO	Left anterior oblique		
LCA	Left coronary artery	VUJ	Vesico-ureteric junction

1

HEAD AND NECK

Q1

a Name the structure labelled A
b Name the structure labelled B
c Name the structure labelled C
d Name the structure labelled D
e Name the structure which fills the space labelled E

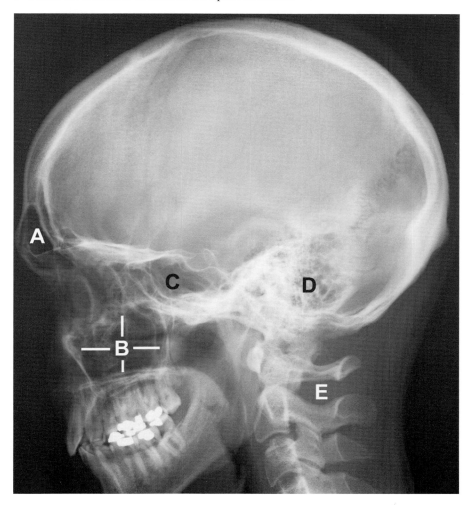

Q2

a Name the structure labelled A
b Name the triangular space labelled B
c Name the structure labelled C
d Name the foramen labelled D
e Name the bony ridge labelled E

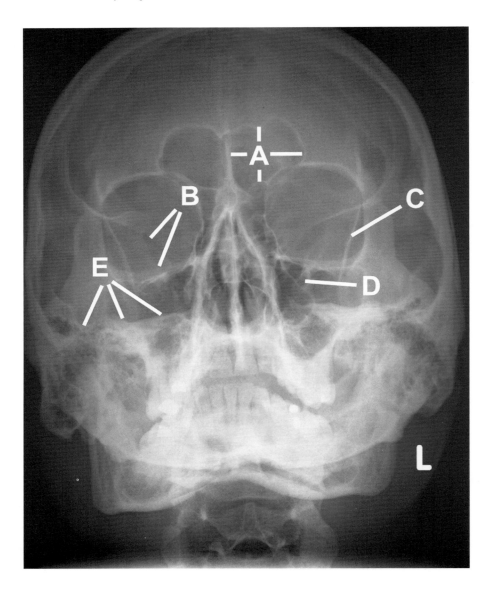

Q3

a Name the structure labelled A
b Name the structure labelled B
c Name the suture labelled C
d Name the structure labelled D
e Name the structure labelled E

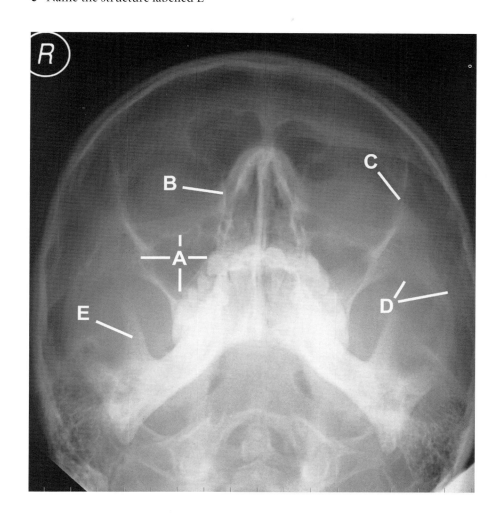

Q4

a Name the skull layer identified with label A
b Name the suture labelled B
c Name the structure that runs along the bony groove identified as C
d Name three structures that pass through D
e Name the structure labelled E

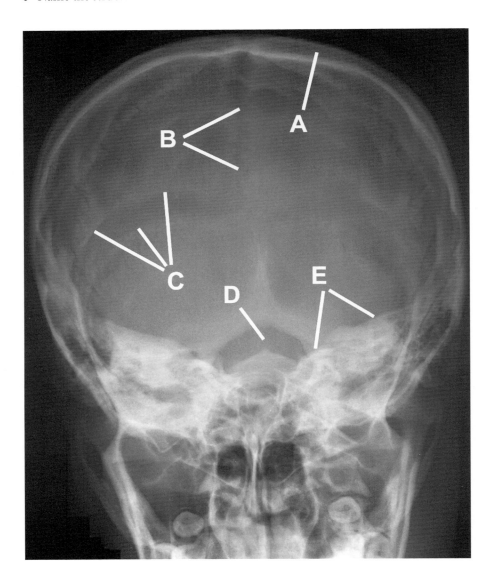

Q5

a Name the structure labelled A
b Name the suture labelled B
c Name the H-shaped suture complex labelled C
d Name the structure labelled D
e Name the suture labelled E

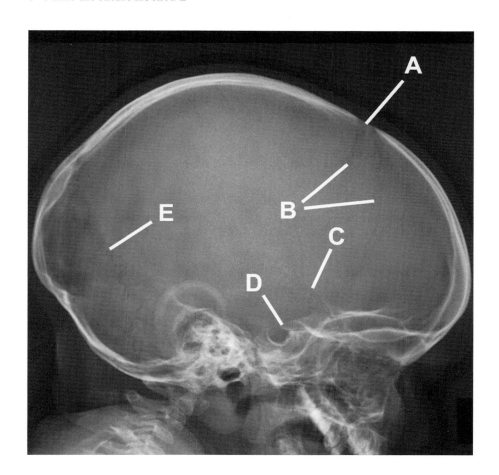

Q6

a Name the structure labelled A
b Name the structure labelled B
c Name all the left upper teeth lying lateral to B
d Name the structure labelled D
e Name the structure labelled E

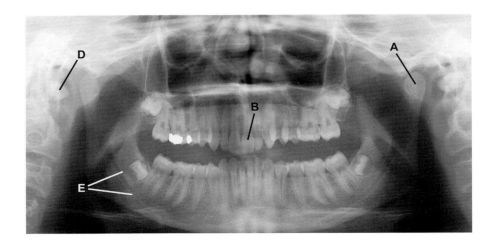

Q7

a Name the most radio-opaque part of the tooth labelled A
b Name the three constituent parts of a tooth as defined by B
c Name the structure labelled C
d Name the structure labelled D
e Name the radiolucent line seen around each tooth below the gumline

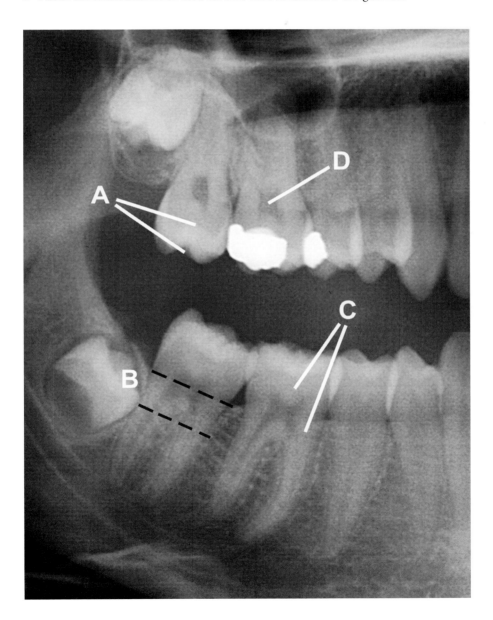

Q8

a Name the foramen labelled A
b Name the foramen labelled B
c Name the foramen labelled C
d Name the structure labelled D
e Name the structure labelled E

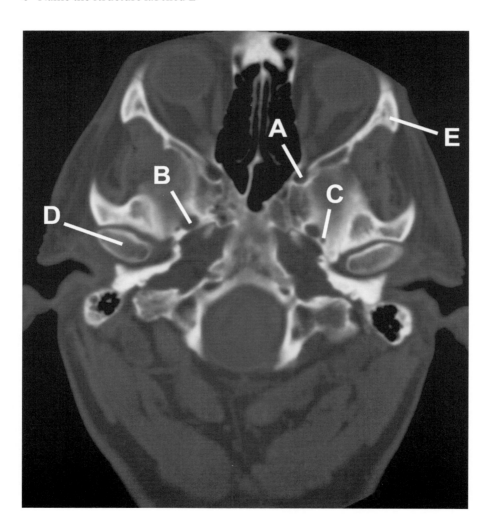

Q9

a Name the structure labelled A
b Name the foramen labelled B
c Name the foramen labelled C
d Name the foramen labelled D
e Name the structure that passes through the foramen labelled E

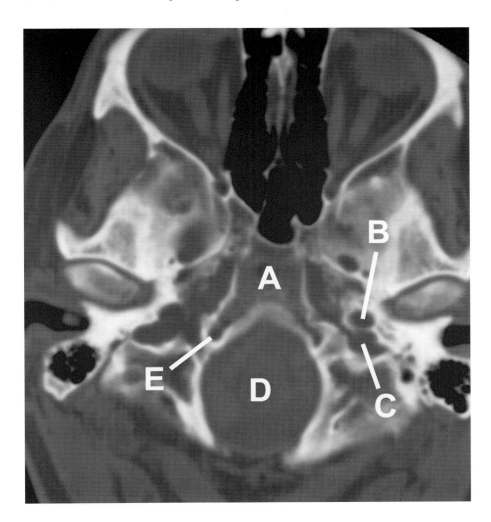

Q10

a Name the bone labelled A
b Name the bony ridge labelled B
c Name the structure labelled C
d Name the structure labelled D
e Name the suture labelled E

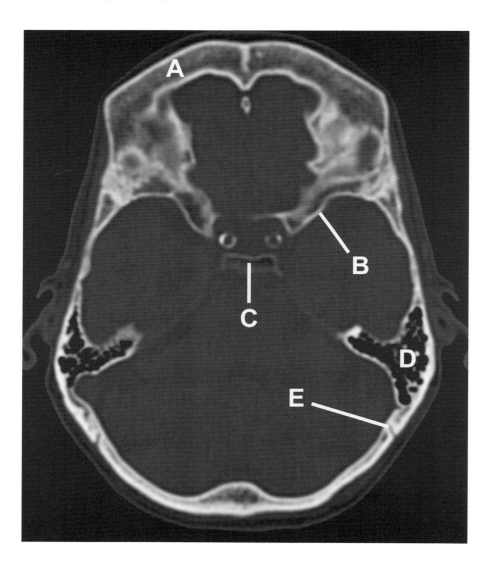

Q11

a Name the structure labelled A
b Name the structure labelled B
c Name the structure labelled C
d Name the structures labelled D
e Name the structure labelled E

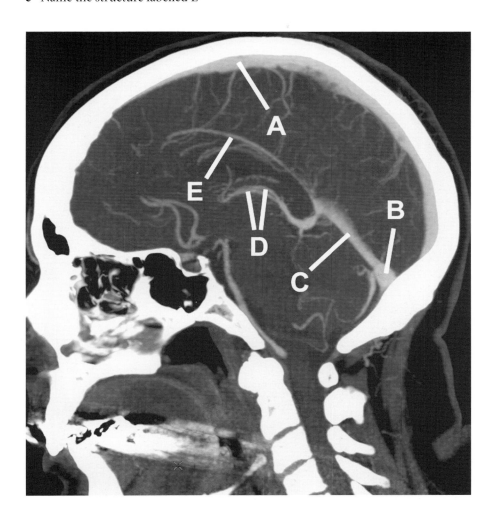

Q12

a Name the artery which supplies the vascular territory indicated by A
b Name the structure labelled B
c Name the structure labelled C
d Name the structure labelled D
e Name the structure labelled E, which has been highlighted with a grey line

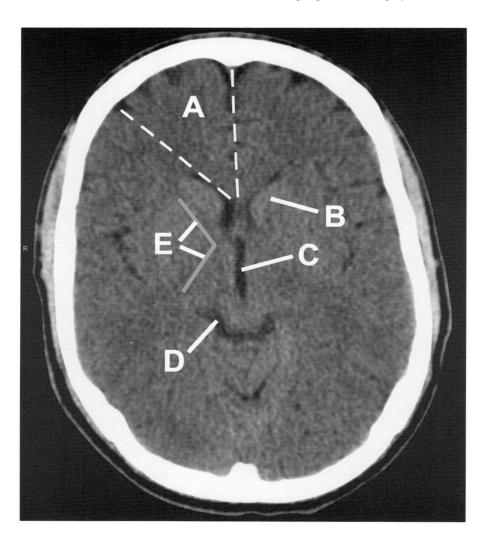

Q13

a Name the fissure labelled A
b Name the CSF space labelled B
c Name the structure labelled C
d Name the structure labelled D
e Name the CSF space labelled E

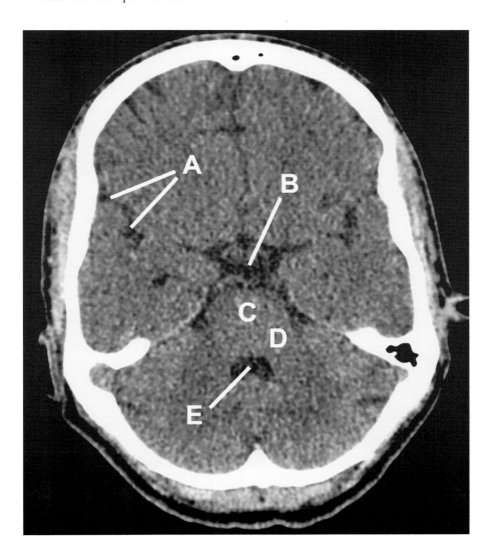

Q14

a Name the structure labelled A
b Name the structure labelled B
c Name the structure labelled C
d Name the structure labelled D
e Name the structure labelled E

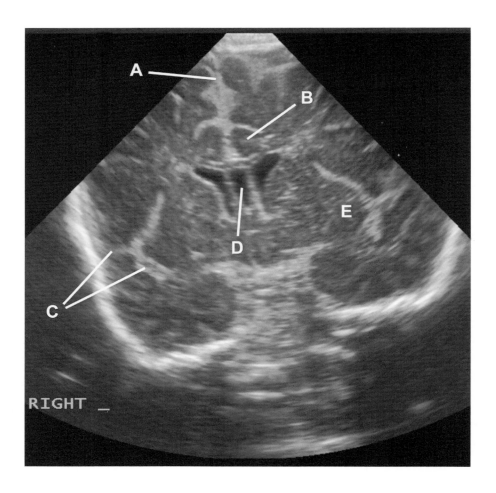

Q15

a Name the structure labelled A

b Name the structure labelled B

c Name the structure labelled C

d Name the space which has been measured

e Describe how blood gets from A to C

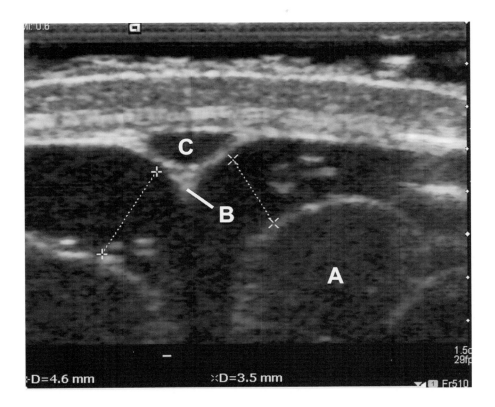

Q16

a Name the structure labelled A
b Name the structure labelled B
c Name the structure labelled C
d Name the structures labelled D
e Name the part of the brainstem demonstrated on this slice

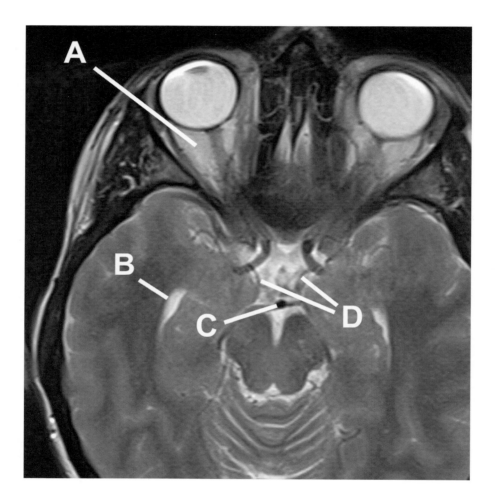

Q17

a Name the structure labelled A
b Name the structure labelled B
c Name the fissure labelled C
d Name the structure labelled D
e Name the structure labelled E

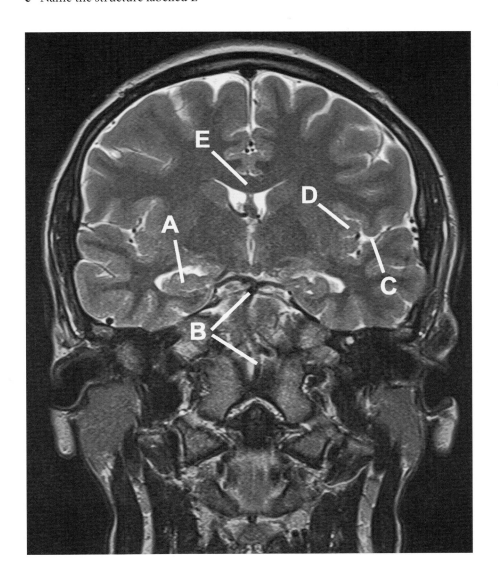

Q18

a Name the constituent parts of the structure labelled A
b Name the structure labelled B
c Name the structure situated between A and B
d Name the structure labelled D
e Name the structure labelled E

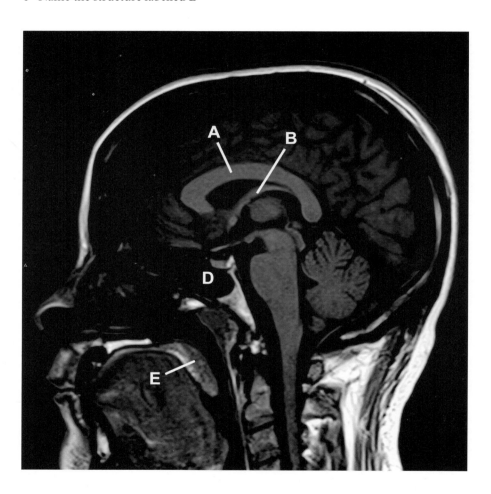

Q19

a Name the structure labelled A
b Name the two structures situated between A and the insular cortex
c Name the CSF channel labelled C
d Name the structure labelled D
e Name the structure labelled E and its two constituent parts

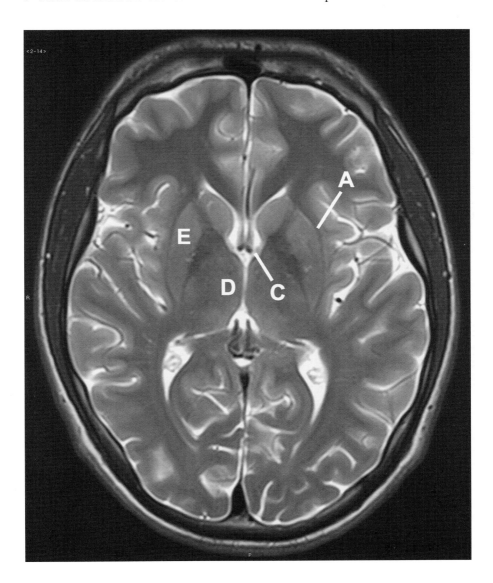

Q20

a Name the structure labelled A
b Name the structure labelled B
c Name the structure labelled C and what it connects
d Name the structures labelled D
e Name the structure labelled E

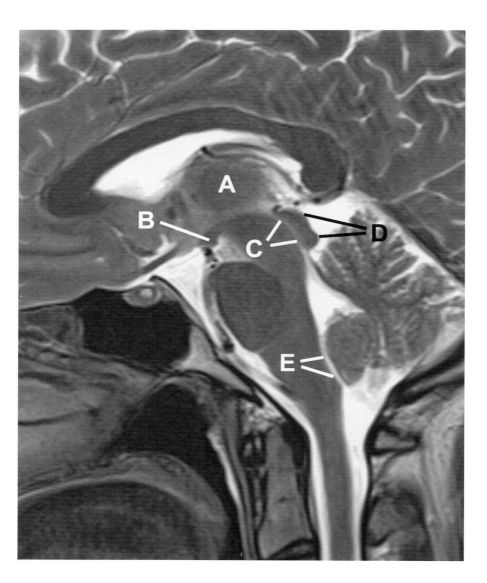

Q21

a Name the structures labelled A
b Name the structure labelled B
c Name the structure labelled C
d Name the structure labelled D
e Name the structures labelled E

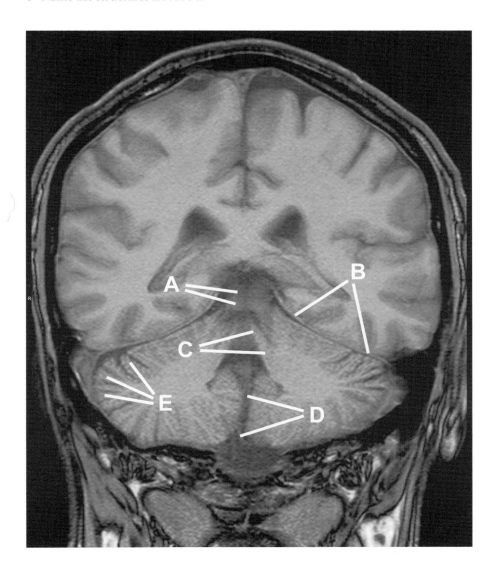

Q22

a Name the structure labelled A
b Name the structure labelled B
c Name the structure labelled C
d Name the structure labelled D
e Name the structure labelled E

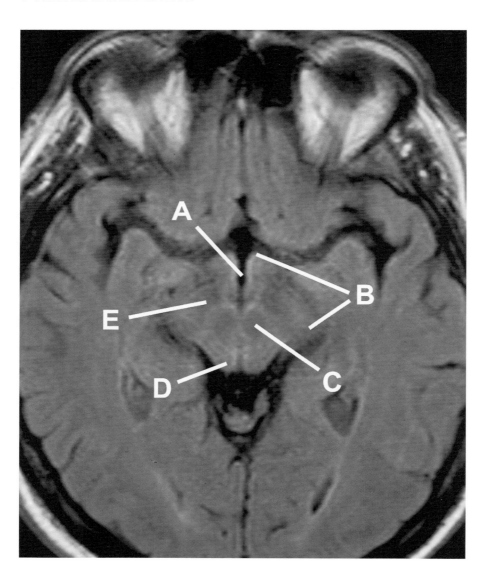

Q23

a Name the structure labelled A
b Name the structure labelled B
c Describe the movement provided by the muscle labelled C
d Name the structure labelled D
e Name the opening labelled E

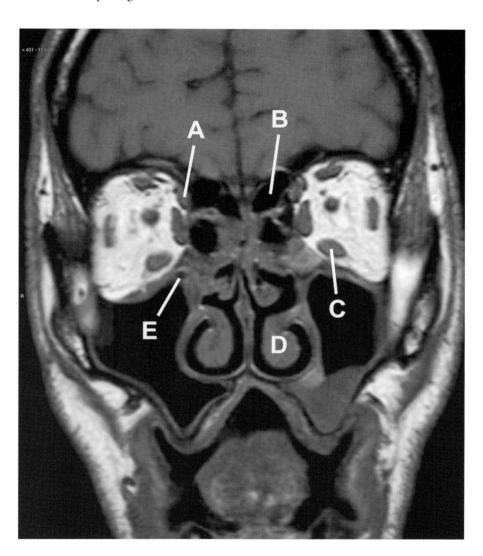

Q24

a Name the structure labelled A
b Name the structure labelled B
c Name the structure labelled C
d Name the CSF filled space containing C in this image
e Name the structure outlined and labelled E

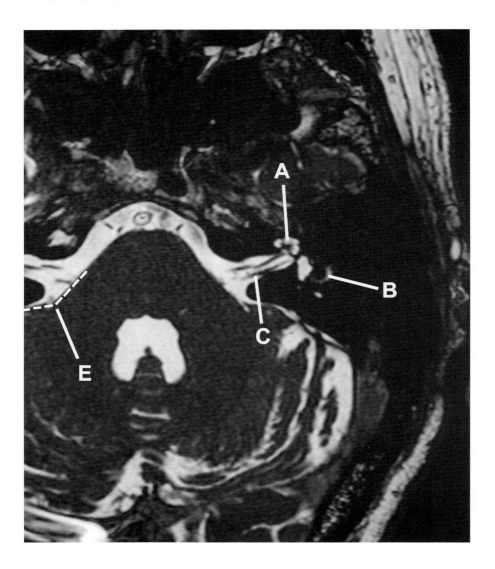

Q25

a Name the structure labelled A
b Name the structure labelled B
c Name the structures labelled C
d Name the structure labelled D
e Name the structure labelled E

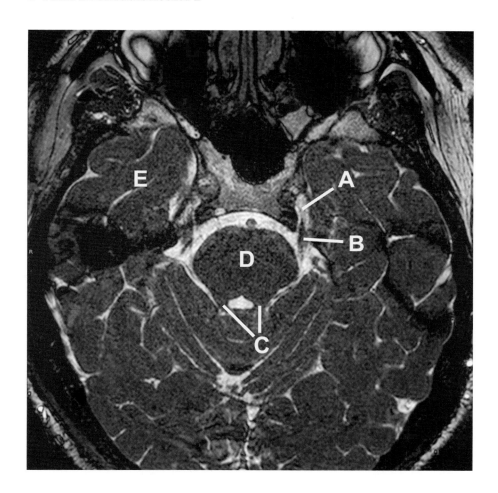

Q26

a Name the vertebral body labelled A
b Name the normal variant demonstrated and labelled as B
c Name the structure outlined by calcification and labelled C
d Name the structure labelled D
e Name the structure labelled E

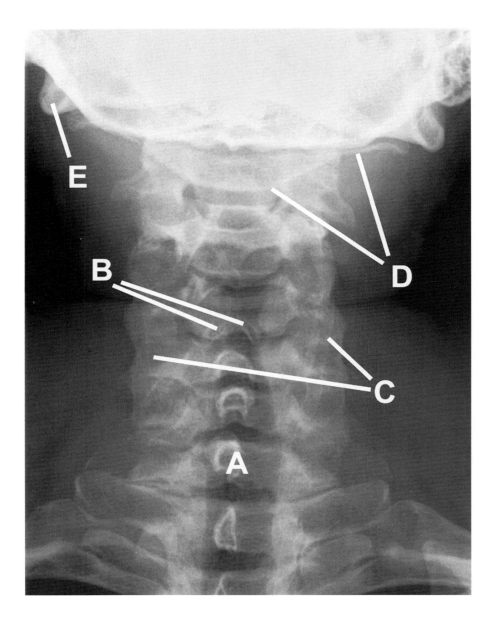

Q27

a Name the upper limit of normal size in adults for the space labelled A
b Name the structures labelled B
c Name the structures labelled C
d Name the structure labelled D
e Name the structure labelled E

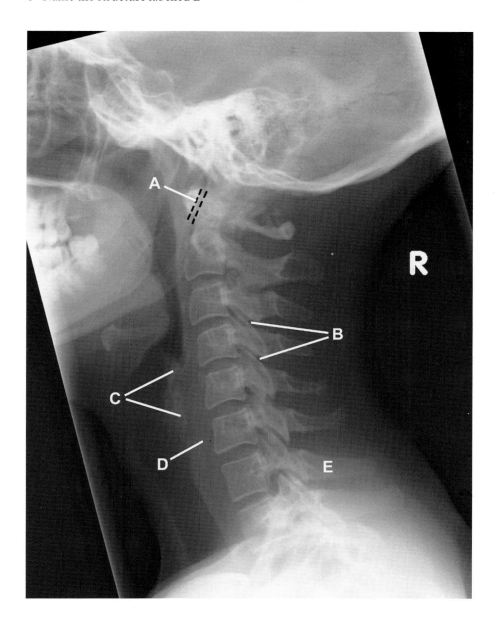

Q28

a Name the structure labelled A
b Name the structure labelled B
c Name the structure labelled C
d Name the structure labelled D
e Name the structure labelled E

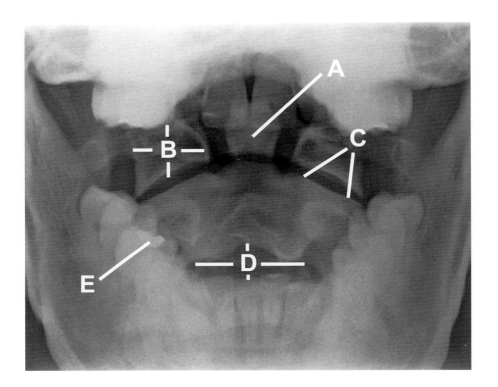

Q29

a Name the structure labelled A
b Name the line labelled B
c Name the inter vertebral space labelled C
d Name the structure labelled D
e Name the structure labelled E

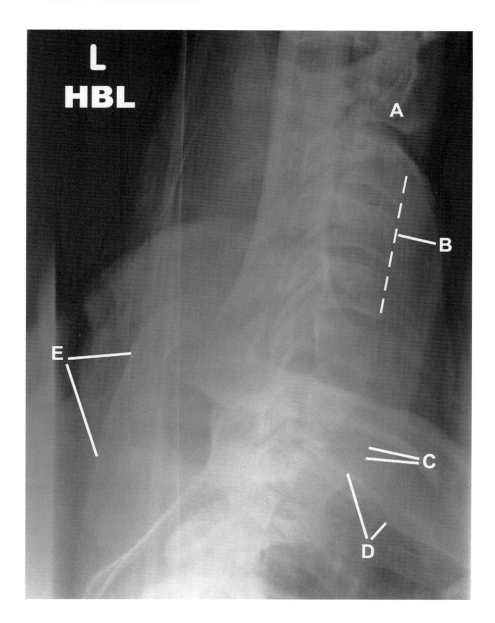

Q30

a Name the structure labelled A
b Name the structures labelled B
c Name the structure labelled C
d Name the major structure that travels through the foramen labelled D
e Name the vertebral level demonstrated

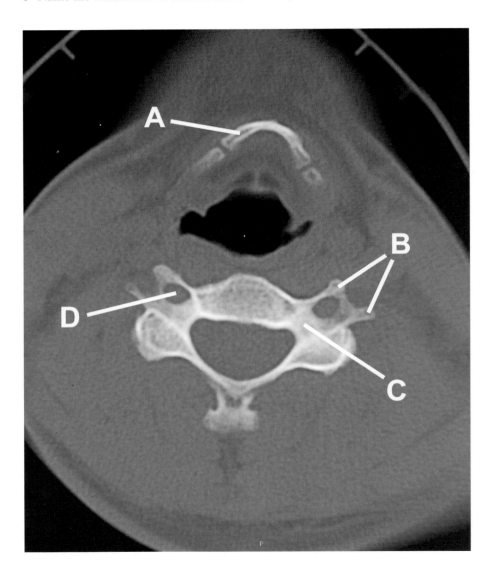

Q31

a Name the structure labelled A
b Name the structure labelled B
c Name the structure labelled C
d Name the structure labelled D
e Name the structure which holds C against A

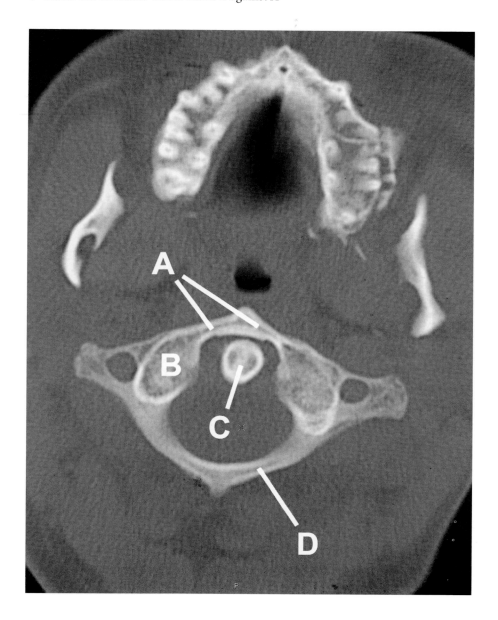

Q32

a Name the structure labelled A
b Name the space labelled B
c Name the muscle labelled C
d Name the space labelled D
e Name the structure labelled E

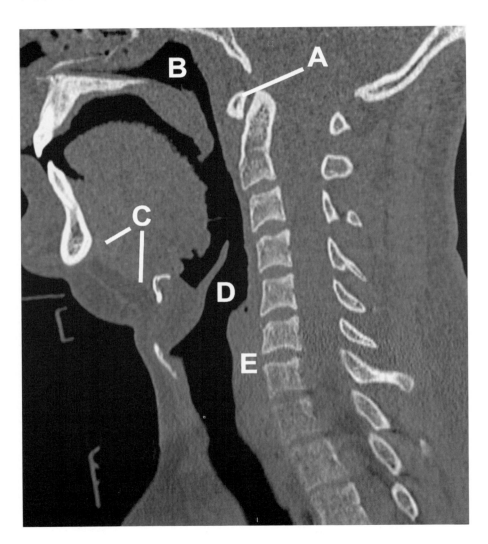

Q33

a Name the structure labelled A
b Name the structure labelled B
c Name the structure labelled C
d Name the structure labelled D
e Name the structures labelled E

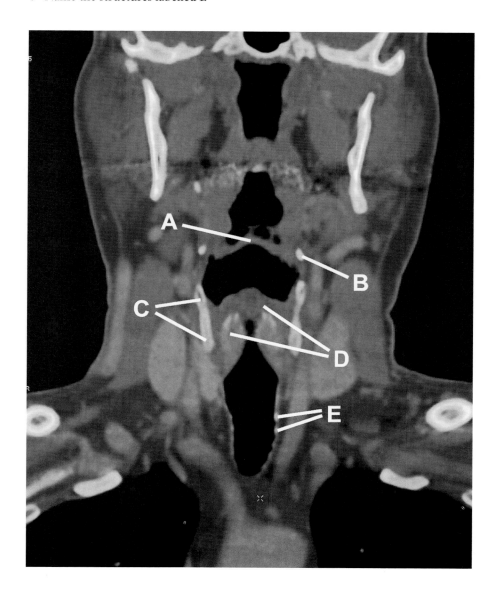

Q34

a Name the structure labelled A
b Name the structure labelled B
c Name the structure labelled C
d Name the echogenic structure labelled D
e Name the constituent part of structure A that passes over structure D

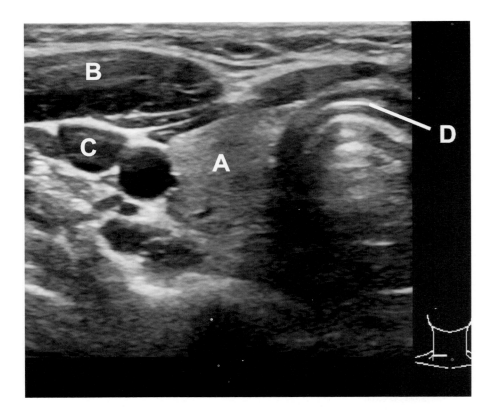

Q35

a Name the structure labelled A
b Name the structure labelled B
c What is the significance of the line drawn and labelled C
d Name the structure labelled D
e Name the structure labelled E

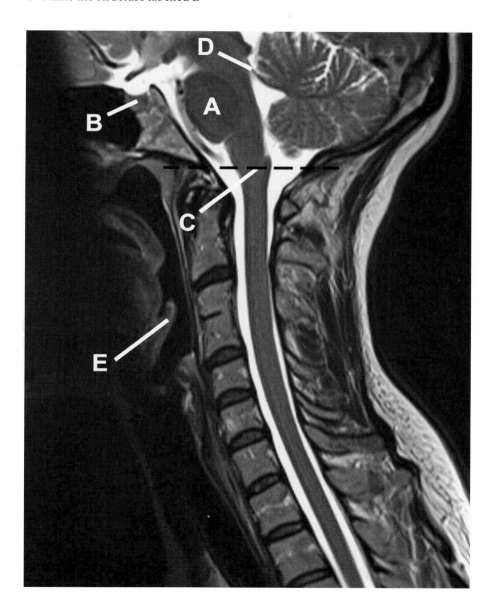

Q36

a Name the structure labelled A
b Name the structure labelled B
c Name the three major structures which pass through the gland labelled C
d Name the structure labelled D
e Name the structure labelled E

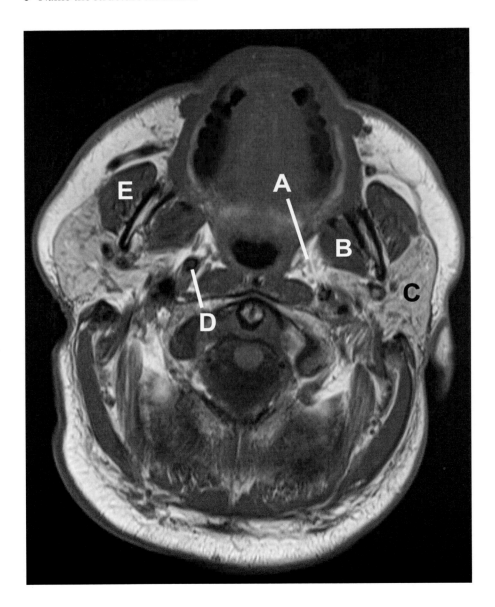

Q37

a Name the cranial nerve that supplies motor function to the structure labelled A
b Name the structure labelled B
c Name the structure labelled C
d Name the structure labelled D
e Name the structure labelled E

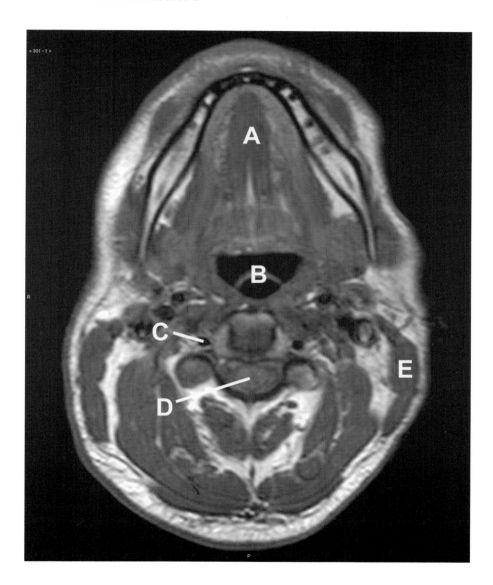

Q38

a Name the structure labelled A
b Name the structure labelled B
c Name the structure labelled C
d Name the osseous structure labelled D
e Name the structure labelled E

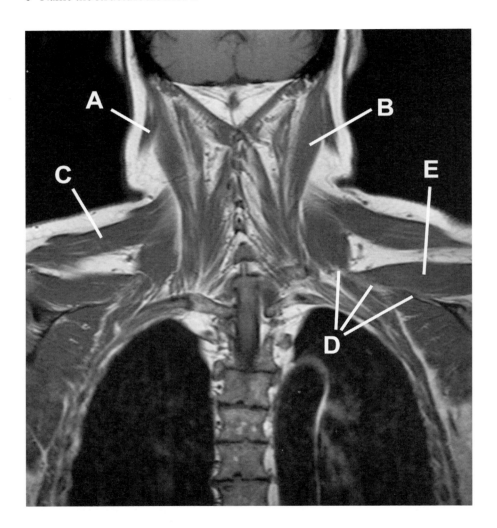

Q39

a Name the structure labelled A
b Name the structures labelled B
c Name the muscle group labelled C
d Name the distal structure to which B contribute
e Describe the relationship between structures B and C within the root of the neck

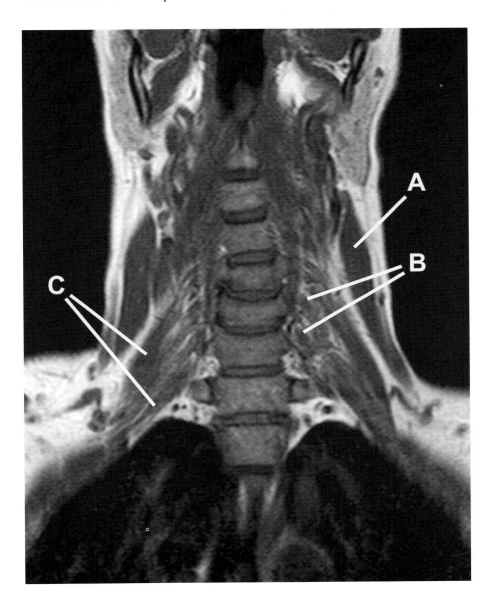

Q40

a Name the structure labelled A
b Name the structure labelled B
c Name three of the commonly described branches of B
d Name the structure through which D passes at the segment labelled
e Name the vessel from which the left common carotid artery arises

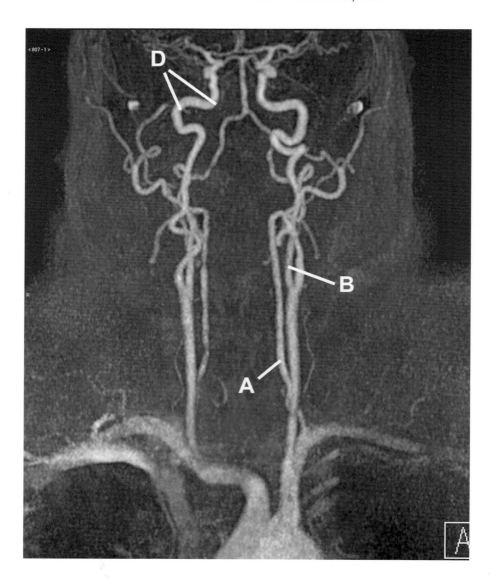

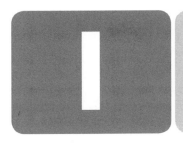

Q1 Answers

a Frontal sinus
b Maxillary sinus
c Sphenoid sinus
d Mastoid air cells
e Interspinous ligament

Radiograph of adult skull, lateral view

The paranasal sinuses should be radiolucent on plain radiography in adults; they can be filled with fluid and/or soft tissue in cases of trauma or disease. In children, the paranasal sinuses are much smaller (maxillary and ethmoidal) or even non-existent (sphenoid and frontal) at birth and progressively pneumatize with age; this is usually complete by the early teen years. The mastoid air cells are normally pneumatized throughout life.

Several ligaments hold the vertebrae together. Most superficially, the supraspinous ligament runs across the tips of the spinous processes and in this region is continuous with the ligamentum nuchae. Deep to this and between adjacent spinous processes lie the interspinous ligaments. Ligamentum flavum covers the internal space between vertebral bodies posteriorly within the spinal canal. The posterior longitudinal ligament runs along the posterior aspect of the vertebral bodies while the anterior longitudinal ligament runs along their anterior aspect.

Scuderi AJ, Harnsberger HR, Boyer RS. Pneumatization of the paranasal sinuses: Normal features of importance to the accurate interpretation of CT scans and MRI images. *Am J Roentgenol* 1993; 160:1101–1104.

Q2 Answers

a Frontal sinus
b Superior orbital fissure
c Innominate line
d Foramen rotundum
e Petrous ridge

Occipito-frontal facial radiograph

This view demonstrates the frontal and ethmoid sinuses well.

Projected within the orbit it is possible to discern the greater and lesser (more medial) wings of sphenoid and the triangular superior orbital fissure in between. The innominate line represents the lateral edge of the greater wing of sphenoid. The foramen rotundum lies beneath the superior orbital fissure.

Q3 Answers

a Maxillary sinus (or antrum)
b Lamina papyracea
c Fronto-zygomatic suture
d Zygomatic arch
e Coronoid process of mandible

Occipito-mental (OM) radiograph

The OM view is used to evaluate the facial bones; it provides excellent visualization of the zygomatic arches and maxillary sinuses. The zygomatic arch is formed via a union of the temporal and zygomatic bones and is said to have the appearance of an elephant's trunk on an OM radiograph. The zygoma forms the prominence of the cheek and it also articulates with the frontal and maxillary bones via appropriately named sutures.

The medial wall represents the thinnest bony part of the orbit and is aptly named the lamina papyracea, meaning paper layer. The ethmoid bone forms most of the medial orbital wall but there are also contributions from the lacrimal, sphenoid and frontal bones.

Q4 Answers

a Diploic layer
b Sagittal suture
c Right transverse venous sinus
d The following all pass through the foramen magnum: junction of medulla and

cervical spinal cord, vertebral arteries, spinal arteries and veins, spinal root of the accessory nerve (CN XI), meninges, menigeal branches of vertebral arteries.

e Petrous ridge

Towne's view (antero-posterior (AP) fronto-occipital projection)

The Towne's view is directed in parallel with the antero-medial skull base and projects the frontal bones over the occipital bones. The facial bones are largely obscured although a Towne's view provides good visualisation of the mandibular condyles.

Skull bones are formed as two parallel layers of cortex surrounding a spongy cancellous layer known as the diploe. Numerous diploic veins connect the intra and extra-cranial vascular spaces.

Q5 Answers

a Anterior fontanelle
b Coronal suture
c Pterion
d Anterior clinoid process
e Lambdoid suture

Skull radiograph in a child of 16 months, lateral view

The skull sutures are unfused in utero, allowing the cranial shape to change during delivery. Antero-superiorly where the coronal suture meets the midline sagittal suture there is initially a defect in bone formation known as the anterior fontanelle. Closure of the anterior fontanelle is variable, but is usually complete by 24 months of age. Where the sagittal suture meets the lamboidal suture posteriorly there is a further defect known as the posterior fontanelle; this usually closes by two months of age. In adulthood, the remnant fontanellae are known anteriorly as the bregma and posteriorly as the lambda.

The weakest point in the adult skull is laterally at the junction of the frontal, temporal, sphenoidal and parietal bones. This H-shaped suture configuration is known as the pterion. Clinically this is important as blunt trauma to this region is more likely to result in fracture and importantly, the middle meningeal artery lies immediately beneath the pterion and can also be damaged.

The paired anterior clinoid processes are a posterior projection from the lesser wing of sphenoid. There are also paired posterior clinoid processes; these arise from the dorsum sellae of the sphenoid bone. The four clinoid processes provide attachment for structures around the pituitary fossa including the diaphragma sellae.

Aisenson MR. Closing of the anterior fontanelle. *Pediatrics* 1950; 6:223–226.

Q6 Answers

a Condylar process of the mandible
b Medial incision, left upper quadrant
c Lateral incisor, canine, 1st and 2nd premolars and 1st, 2nd and 3rd molars (3rd is unerupted)
d Anterior arch of C1
e Mandibular canal

Orthopantomogram (OPG)

The OPG provides a single image of the entire dentition, lower maxilla and mandible. This is achieved through a form of tomography where the image is taken whilst moving round the patient. In addition to the structures described, an OPG also usually shows the anterior aspect of the upper cervical spine, maxillary sinuses, nasal septum and hyoid (all seen on this image).

Adult teeth number 32 (20 deciduous teeth in childhood) and are usually divided into quadrants of eight for descriptive purposes (left and right upper and lower). In each quadrant there is a medial and lateral incisor, a canine, two premolars and three molars. The third molar may remain unerupted well into adulthood (wisdom teeth).

The mandibular canal carries the inferior alveolar artery and nerve (a branch of CN V_3) which exit the mandible via the mental foramen (not shown here).

Q7 Answers

a Enamel
b Crown, neck and root
c Dentine
d Pulp cavity
e Periodontal membrane

Radiograph of upper and lower right teeth in an adult, zoomed up image

Each tooth is composed of a crown (above the gumline), a neck and a root. Teeth are primarily formed from dentine which is similar to compact bone. The inner core of a tooth is composed of soft tissues (and is therefore more radiolucent) and is known as the pulp cavity. Beneath the gumline, the division between tooth and surrounding bone is highlighted by the very dense bone of the lamina dura lying immediately outside the radiolucent line of the periodontal membrane of the tooth. The intra-oral part of each tooth (crown) is covered by dense radio-opaque enamel which is the hardest part of the tooth. Defects to the enamel (usually as a consequence of decay) are repaired with dental fillings; these are dense and appear radio-opaque on radiography (as shown).

Q8 Answers

a Foramen rotundum
b Foramen ovale
c Foramen spinosum
d Condylar process of the mandible
e Frontal process of the zygoma

CT with bone windows at level of skull base, axial section

The skull base is generally symmetrical across the midline sagittal plane and its many foramina are clearly visible on CT. On each side, the foramen rotundum (more rounded appearance than foramen ovale) transmits the second (maxillary) branch of the trigeminal nerve (CN V). Postero-lateral to this, the foramen ovale transmits the third (mandibular) division of the trigeminal nerve. Immediately postero-lateral again sits the foramen spinosum; this allows passage of the middle meningeal artery (a branch of the maxillary artery).

Q9 Answers

a Clivus
b Carotid canal
c Jugular foramen
d Foramen magnum
e Hypoglossal nerve

CT with bone windows at level of skull base, axial section

The clivus represents the posterior aspect of the sphenoid bone and forms part of the anterior wall of the posterior cranial fossa. The pons sits immediately posterior to the clivus.

The carotid artery takes a tortuous course through the skull base; it enters the skull via the carotid canal traversing the foramen lacerum (seen on this image just medial to the carotid canal as a ragged opening) to enter the cranial cavity. Immediately thereafter, the carotid artery enters the venous cavernous sinus where it makes several turns before entering the subarachnoid space to divide into its terminal branches.

In addition to the jugular vein, the jugular foramen transmits cranial nerves IX (glossopharyngeal), X (vagus) and XI (accessory). The hypoglossal canal lies medial to and below the jugular foramen and transmits the hypoglossal nerve (CN XII). The foramen magnum is the major and only unpaired opening in the cranial floor and allows the medulla to continue caudally as the spinal cord. In addition, the vertebral arteries enter the skull via this route along with the spinal root of CN XI.

Q10 Answers

a Frontal bone
b Lesser wing of sphenoid
c Dorsum sellae
d Mastoid air cells
e Lambdoidal suture

CT with bone windows showing cranial fossae, axial section

The cranium is divided into three fossae which are arranged in a stepwise fashion from front to back. The anterior cranial fossa, containing the frontal lobes of the cerebral hemispheres, is at the highest level and lies between the frontal bones anteriorly and the sphenoid ridge (formed by the lesser wing of sphenoid) posteriorly. The base of the anterior cranial fossa is predominantly formed by the orbital plates of the frontal bones separating the frontal lobes of the brain from the orbits. In the midline the perforated cribriform plates of the ethmoid bone enable olfactory nerve fibres to pass from the nasal cavity to the olfactory bulbs. The floor of the middle cranial fossa is formed anteriorly by the greater wing of sphenoid and posteriorly by the petrous part of the temporal bone; the petrous ridge defines its posterior limit. The middle cranial fossa supports the anterior aspect of the temporal lobes. The posterior cranial fossa is formed largely by the occipital bone and contains the cerebellum.

The dorsum sellae is the posterior part of the bony cavity formed to house the pituitary gland and arises from the body of the sphenoid bone.

It is important to recognize the various skull sutures and their normal locations as fractures can have similar appearances.

Q11 Answers

a Superior sagittal sinus
b Confluence of sinuses
c Straight sinus
d Internal cerebral veins
e Inferior sagittal sinus

CT venogram, maximum intensity projection, midline sagittal view

The dural venous sinuses exist between the two layers of dura and allow drainage of blood from the brain. Superficial cerebral veins coalesce into larger vessels (e.g. the superior anastomotic vein of Trolard, and the inferior anastomotic vein of Labbe) and then tend to drain via the superior sagittal or transverse sinuses. Deep cerebral veins such as the internal cerebral veins coalesce to form the great cerebral vein (of Galen) which combines with the inferior sagittal sinus to form the straight sinus. The superior sagittal sinus combines with the straight sinus at the confluence of sinuses. From here, venous blood drains via the transverse sinuses (one side is usually dominant and therefore larger), through the sigmoid sinuses and into the internal jugular veins bilaterally. Anteriorly, venous blood from the ophthalmic and superficial middle cerebral veins as well as from the sphenoparietal sinus collects in the cavernous sinuses. The cavernous sinuses are situated on either side of the body of sphenoid and each contains the first intracranial part of the internal carotid artery and the abducent nerve (CN VI). The occulomotor (CN III), trochlear (CN IV), plus ophthalmic and maxillary branches of the trigeminal nerve (CN V) course through the lateral wall of the cavernous sinuses. Blood ultimately drains from the cavernous sinuses through the superior and inferior petrosal sinuses. The superior petrosal runs along the anterior margin of the tentorium cerebelli at the petrous ridge to reach the distal transverse sinus where it continues as the sigmoid sinus. The inferior petrosal drains more inferiorly joining the distal sigmoid sinus as it becomes the internal jugular vein.

Q12 Answers

a Anterior cerebral artery
b Head of the caudate
c Third ventricle
d Ambient cistern
e Internal capsule

CT brain scan, axial section at the level of the third ventricle

Vascular territories of the brain are best demonstrated diagrammatically; an in-depth description is beyond the scope of this text.

The caudate nucleus is a long thin structure with a head, body and tail. Its course is compliant with that of the lateral ventricle. The caudate is composed of grey matter and is considered one of the basal ganglia which as a group are concerned with movement as part of the extra-pyramidal system.

Cerebrospinal fluid (CSF) is produced through ultrafiltration of blood plasma by choroid plexus; most is produced in the lateral ventricles. CSF flows from the lateral ventricles to the midline third ventricle through the interventricular foramina (of Monro); from here it passes through the midbrain via the cerebral aqueduct to the fourth ventricle posteriorly. Once in the fourth ventricle, CSF will pass either to the sub-arachnoid space (predominantly) via the medial and lateral apertures of Magendie and Luschka, respectively, or in a caudal direction through the central canal of the spinal cord. The named ventricles and several subarachnoid cisterns are visible on CT. The ambient cisterns extend around both sides of the midbrain and communicate posteriorly with the quadrigeminal cistern. The posterior cerebral arteries pass through the ambient cisterns.

The internal capsule represents white matter tracts connecting the cerebral cortices with the brainstem and spinal cord. The anterior and posterior limbs meet at the genu (meaning knee) and form a V shape which is visible on axial CT slices. Both primary motor and sensory pathways for the entire body are concentrated in the anterior two thirds of the posterior limb; the upper body is represented anteriorly towards the genu while the lower body is represented more posteriorly.

Q13 Answers

a Sylvian fissure
b Pontine/interpeduncular cistern
c Pons
d Middle cerebellar peduncle
e Fourth ventricle

Contrast enhanced CT head, axial section at the level of the fourth ventricle

The sylvian fissure (or lateral sulcus) separates the frontal and temporal lobes and contains branches of the middle cerebral artery. The pontine cistern is continuous with the interpeduncular cistern above and the foramen magnum below and contains the basilar artery. Due to the angulation of this CT image (parallel with skull base) the CSF space shown contains elements of both pontine and interpeduncular cisterns.

The pons is recognizable by its anterior bulge ('pot belly' appearance when seen in sagittal section) and by the largest of the cerebellar peduncles (middle) connecting it posteriorly with the cerebellum (also forming the lateral walls of the fourth ventricle).

Q14 Answers

a Interhemispheric fissure containing falx cerebri
b Cingulate gyrus
c Sylvian fissure
d Cavum septum pellucidum
e Insular cortex

Ultrasound of neonatal brain, coronal section

Prior to closure of the anterior fontanelle it is possible to visualize the neonatal brain using ultrasound.

The two cerebral hemispheres meet in the midline and are separated by the interhemispheric (great longitudinal) fissure. The falx cerebri is a double dural layer running through this fissure connecting the superior and inferior sagittal venous sinuses. The inferior border of the interhemispheric fissure is bounded by the corpus callosum. The first major gyrus superior to and running parallel with the corpus callosum (best seen on sagittal view) is the cingulate gyrus. Functionally the cingulate gyri are part of the limbic system.

Cavum septum pellucidum is a normal variant where CSF is found between the septi pellucidum in the midline. The insular cortex lies deep to the sylvian fissure (or lateral sulcus).

Q15 Answers

a Cerebral hemisphere, frontal/parietal lobe
b Origin of falx cerebri
c Superior sagittal sinus
d Subarachnoid space
e Superficial cerebral veins drain to the superior sagittal sinus

Ultrasound of neonatal brain, coronal section with close up view of subarachnoid space

As part of the assessment of the neonatal brain using ultrasound, the subarachnoid spaces are measured. The subarachnoid space is filled with CSF and surrounds the brain. Multiple bridging cerebral veins cross the subarachnoid space and drain into the venous sinuses. The arachnoid layer is usually closely adherent to the more superficial dura. Only a *potential* space exists between these layers; however this potential space can become real if the bridging cerebral veins are damaged leading to a subdural haemorrhage. The third meningeal layer is the pia and it is closely adherent to the brain surface and separated from the arachnoid layer by the aforementioned CSF filling the subarachnoid space.

Q16 Answers

a Intra-conal fat
b Temporal (inferior) horn of the right lateral ventricle
c Basilar artery
d Posterior communicating arteries
e Midbrain

T2W MRI of head, axial section

The extra-ocular muscles are arranged as a cone; this configuration is used to define intra and extra-conal compartments within the orbit.

The circle of Willis supplies arterial blood to the brain and is formed when the basilar and the right and left internal carotid arteries divide at the base of the brain. The basilar divides to form right and left posterior cerebral arteries, while each internal carotid divides to form an anterior and a middle cerebral artery. Posterior communicating arteries link the posterior and middle cerebral vessels bilaterally while the anterior communicating artery completes the circle (of Willis) by connecting the two anterior cerebral arteries. This configuration of anastomoses between the anterior and posterior arterial blood supplies to the brain provides the potential for collateral flow if part of the circulation is compromised.

The midbrain can be recognized in axial cross section by identification of the two cerebral peduncles anteriorly which are separated by the interpeduncular cistern. Posteriorly the midbrain has four rounded prominences, the superior and inferior colliculi (also known as the corpora quadrigemini).

Q17 Answers

a Hippocampus
b Basilar artery
c Sylvian fissure
d Insula
e Corpus callosum

T2W MRI of brain, coronal section at level of the hippocampi

The limbic system describes a number of structures including the hippocampus, amygdala, cingulate gyrus, mammillary body and fornix (to name only a few) which are grouped as two C-shaped arches located medially in the cerebral hemispheres. They are functionally related, all being involved with emotion, memory and instinctive behaviour. Many of these structures are recognizable on MRI. The hippocampus is best seen in the coronal plane as a curved elevation in the floor of the inferior horn of the lateral ventricle. The parahippocampal gyrus lies inferior to the hippocampus and forms the infero-medial part of the temporal lobe. The insular cortex forms the floor of the lateral sulcus (sylvian fissure); its function is not clearly defined but is related to the limbic system.

The corpus callosum is the largest of the commissural white matter tracts (commisures link corresponding parts of the two hemispheres) and is best demonstrated on a midline sagittal view.

Q18 Answers

a Rostrum, genu, body and splenium of the corpus callosum
b Fornix
c Septum pellucidum
d Sphenoid sinus
e Soft palate

TW1 MRI, midline sagittal section

The corpus callosum is the largest of the commissural white matter tracts. The genu (or knee) is the bend at its anterior end. Inferior to the genu is the rostrum, posterior to the genu running horizontally is the body of the corpus callosum, while the splenium is its bulbous posterior part.

The fornices are white matter tracts which run from the hippocampi postero-laterally to converge on the thalamus anteriorly near the midline.

Between the corpus callosum and the fornices lies the septi pellucidum. These paper thin structures form the medial wall of the lateral ventricles. Often the two septi pellucidum are opposed anteriorly in the midline; if there is a CSF filled space between them it is known as cavum septum pellucidum.

Of the four paired paranasal sinuses, the sphenoid and frontal sinuses are visible in the midline.

The roof of the oral cavity is known as the palate and is composed of hard and soft parts. The hard palate is formed by the palatine processes of the maxillae and the paired palatine bones and composes the anterior two thirds of the palate. The soft palate is a mobile fibro-muscular continuation of the hard palate which prevents food from passing up into the nasal cavity during swallowing.

Q19 Answers

a External capsule
b Claustrum and extreme capsule
c Foramen of Monro
d Thalamus
e Lentiform nucleus composed of globus pallidus and putamen

T2W MRI of brain at level of third ventricle, axial section

The internal capsule is a white matter tract and forms a V-shape on axial section with the point directed towards the midline. Medial to the anterior limb of this V is the head of the caudate nucleus while the thalamus lies medial to the posterior limb and lateral to the third ventricle. Lateral to the internal capsule on this view is the lentiform nucleus. Like the caudate nucleus, the lentiform nucleus is one of the paired basal ganglia which as a group are functionally involved with movement. The lentiform is lens-shaped when viewed on axial section, hence the name. The constituent parts of the lentiform nucleus are (from medial to lateral) globus pallidus and putamen. The external capsule is a further white matter tract lying lateral to the lentiform nucleus. Lateral to the external capsule, in order, are the claustrum (further paired basal ganglia), the extreme capsule and finally the insular cortex.

Q20 Answers

a Massa intermedia of thalamus
b Mamillary body
c Cerebral aqueduct (of Sylvius) allows CSF to flow from 3rd to 4th ventricles
d Superior and inferior colliculi
e Median aperture (of Magendie)

T2W MRI of brain zoomed up image, midline sagittal section

The massa intermedia connects the left and right thalami in the midline. CSF within the third ventricle flows around the massa intermedia within the third ventricle.

The mamillary bodies are part of the limbic system and connect with the fornices bilaterally. The mamillary bodies are in the roof of the interpeduncular cistern.

The colliculi are paired as two superior and two inferior. They form four masses of tissue situated as the corners of a square on the posterior aspect of the tectal plate of the midbrain. Functionally, the colliculi are concerned with reflexes by acting as relay pathways; the superior relate to vision, the inferior to hearing.

Q21 Answers

a Superior and inferior colliculus
b Tentorium cerebelli
c Left superior cerebellar peduncle
d Vermis
e Folia

T1W MRI through cerebellum and 4th ventricle, coronal section

The cerebellum lies in the posterior fossa of the cranium and is separated from the cerebral hemispheres by the tentorium cerebelli, an invagination of dura between the cerebral and cerebellar hemispheres similar to the falx cerebri in the sagittal midline. The cerebellum lies posterior to the brain stem and the two are connected by three paired peduncles, named superior, middle and inferior. Between these peduncles and between the cerebellum and brainstem is the 4th ventricle. The two cerebellar hemispheres are joined in the midline by the vermis. Each hemisphere is divided into anterior, posterior and flocculonodular (inferior) lobes; the nodule lies at the end of the vermis near the floor of the 4th ventricle. The cerebellar surface is highly convoluted, the gyri are known as folia (as in foliage or leaves).

Q22 Answers

a Interpeduncular cistern
b Crus cerebri
c Red nucleus
d Superior colliculus
e Substantia nigra

T1W MRI at level of midbrain, axial section

The crus cerebri are white matter tracts that run from the internal capsule to the pons over the antero-lateral aspect of the midbrain. The cerebral peduncle is the whole of the midbrain excluding the tectum (superior and inferior colliculi). A CSF cleft is formed between the paired cerebral peduncles anteriorly known as the interpeduncular cistern; occult subarachnoid haemorrhage can sometimes be found here.

The red nuclei and substantia nigra are both concerned with motor function; the substantia nigra is considered one of the basal ganglia. The red nuclei are usually found at the level of the superior colliculi.

The cerebral aqueduct (of Sylvius) may be seen on an axial section of midbrain between the red nuclei and superior colliculus as an area of CSF signal intensity (this is just visible on the image provided).

Q23 Answers

a Superior oblique muscle
b Posterior ethmoid sinus
c The inferior rectus muscle provides downward (and medial) rotation of the eyeball
d Inferior nasal concha (or turbinate)
e Maxillary ostium (part of the ostiomeatal complex)

TIW MRI through posterior orbits and paranasal sinuses

The eye moves through the function of six muscles. These are named superior, inferior, medial and lateral rectus and the superior and inferior oblique muscles. The recti muscles pull the eye in the direction they are situated. The oblique muscles are named counter intuitively as the superior depresses the eye while the inferior raises it. Most of these muscles are supplied by the occulomotor nerve (CN III), except the lateral rectus and superior oblique which are supplied by the abducent (CN VI) and trochlear nerves (CN IV), respectively.

The three paired nasal conchae (superior, middle and inferior) are separated by spaces known as meati. The paranasal sinuses are situated around the nasal cavity and also drain into it. They are paired and include the frontal, ethmoid (with anterior, middle and posterior parts), sphenoid and maxillary sinuses. The maxillary sinus drains from its superior medial aspect via the maxillary ostium into the ethmoid infundibulum which in turn drains into the middle meatus of the nasal cavity. These structures are collectively known as the ostiomeatal complex. The nasolacrimal duct running from the medial angle of the eye also drains into the nasal cavity (inferior meatus).

Q24 Answers

a Cochlea
b Lateral (or horizontal) semicircular canal
c Vestibular nerve (superior or inferior)
d Internal auditory meatus
e Cerebello-pontine angle

T2W MRI of middle ear structures, zoomed up high resolution axial section

Structures in the internal auditory meatus (IAM) can be well visualized on high resolution T2W MRI scans (using IAM specific sequences, e.g. CISS (constructive interface in steady state).

Four nerves run through the IAM and depending on the level of the axial section are usually visualized as two superior and two inferior nerves running in parallel. With a more superiorly orientated section, the facial nerve is seen anterior to the superior division of the vestibular nerve (CN VII and one of the three branches of CN VIII, respectively). With a slightly inferiorly orientated section the cochlear nerve is seen anterior to the inferior division of the vestibular nerve (both branches of CN VIII, the vestibulocochlear nerve). This orientation may be difficult to appreciate on axial section as the superior and inferior nerves lie very close together (the two anterior nerves seem to cross over on the image provided). For identification purposes, remember that the vestibular nerves lie posterior to the facial and cochlear nerves. To ease orientation and identification of the individual nerves, images can be reformatted and viewed in an oblique sagittal section. In this scenario the nerves are orientated as the four corners of a square.

The cochlea lie antero-medial to the semicircular canals within the petrous portion of the temporal bone.

There are three semicircular canals; anterior, posterior and lateral. The lateral (or horizontal) canal is orientated in-plane with an axial section; the other two are orientated vertically with respect to the horizontal canal and at 90 degrees to one another. The posterior canal runs in parallel with the petrous ridge, while the anterior canal lies at 90 degrees to the petrous ridge.

Q25 Answers

a Meckel's cave
b Trigeminal nerve
c Superior cerebellar peduncles
d Pons
e Anterior temporal lobe

The trigeminal nerve (CN V) arises from the pons and passes anteriorly into Meckel's cave where it forms the trigeminal ganglion. Meckel's cave is a CSF filled space lined by dura which lies postero-lateral to the cavernous sinus on the antero-medial aspect of the petrous temporal bone.

The superior cerebellar peduncles arise from the midbrain but run infero-posterioly and are therefore visualized on this oblique view through the upper pons.

Kamel HAM and Toland J. Trigeminal Nerve Anatomy: Illustrated Using Examples of Abnormalities. *Am J Roentgenol* 2001; 176:247–251.

Q26 Answers

a   C7 vertebra
b   Bifid spinous process of C4 vertebra
c   Thyroid cartilage
d   Hyoid bone
e   Angle of mandible

Radiograph of C-spine, AP view

Individual vertebrae can be distinguished on an AP cervical radiograph by counting up from T1, which is the first to articulate with a rib (bear in mind C7 can sometimes articulate with a normal variant cervical rib, but this is usually much shorter than the typical upper thoracic ribs). Often, the dens of C2 is also visible and enables vertebral identification from the top.

The laryngeal cartilages can calcify with age and this makes their identification on plain radiography possible. The thyroid cartilage is the largest of the laryngeal cartilages. Each lamina of the thyroid cartilage lies antero-lateral to the vocal cords and their associated cartilages, providing protection and support. These laminae slope outwards from below as shown and meet in the midline at the laryngeal prominence (also known as Adam's apple). The thyroid cartilage is connected to the hyoid bone above via the thyrohyoid membrane and to the cricoid cartilage below via the cricothyroid ligament. It is the top free edge of the cricothyroid membrane that forms the vocal cord. In the mid-line running between the arch of the cricoid and the inferior aspect of the thyroid cartilage is a thickening of the cricothyroid membrane called the cricothyroid ligament.

The hyoid bone divides the neck into infra and supra-hyoid regions and provides anchorage for a number of muscles in the anterior neck. The hyoid is active during swallowing and speech.

Q27 Answers

a 3mm
b Zygapophyseal (facet) joint spaces
c Calcification within laryngeal cartilages
d Prevertebral soft tissues
e Spinous process of C7 (vertebra prominens)

Radiograph of neck, lateral view

The distance between the anterior arch of C1 and the dens of C2 should be less than 3mm in adults and can be up to 5mm in children. Disruption of the joint may be indicated by widening of this space.

The cervical spine is more mobile than other parts of the vertebral column; the obliquely orientated superior and inferior facets allow rotation, flexion/extension and lateral bending. Facet joints are also known as zygapophyseal joints. On a true lateral view, the facet joints should run in parallel with one another.

The prevertebral soft tissues of the neck usually measure only a few millimetres anterior to the vertebral bodies of C1–4. Below this level the prevertebral layer expands (primarily due to the oesophagus) and when measured is usually equivalent in size to the corresponding vertebral body. Another way to remember this is with the phrase '7 at 2 and 2 at 7'; this translates as 7mm of soft tissue at the C2 level and 2cm of soft tissue at the C7 level. Trauma, infection and malignancy can all enlarge the prevertebral soft tissue.

The spinous process of C7 is the largest of all cervical vertebrae and so is also named vertebra prominens; this may be useful when trying to identify a particular vertebra if the provided views are limited.

Q28 Answers

a Dens (odontoid peg) of C2
b Lateral mass of C1
c Superior articular facet of C2
d C2–3 interspace
e Reparative 'filling' in left lower molar tooth

Radiograph of odontoid peg, AP open mouth view

With an open mouth view, the dens of C2 is seen to lie centrally between the two lateral masses of C1. The vertebral body and spinous process of C2 are also usually seen. There is some overlap from the dentition and mandible on this view; these features should be recognized.

Q29 Answers

a Body of C2 vertebra
b Anterior vertebral line
c C7/T1 joint (interspace)
d 1st rib
e Posterior border of the scapula

Radiograph of cervical and upper thoracic spine, lateral 'swimmers' view

On a lateral c-spine radiograph, overlap of the shoulders can restrict visualization of the C7/T1 joint. The swimmers view places the patient with one arm up and the other down (as if in mid stroke of front crawl or freestyle) to minimize this bony overlap.

Several vertical lines can be used to assess spinal alignment including the anterior vertebral line which joins the anterior aspects of the vertebral bodies.

It is important to recognize the other overlapping bony contours seen on this view such as the humerus, scapula, clavicle and ribs.

Q30 Answers

a Body of hyoid bone
b Tubercles (anterior and posterior) of left transverse process
c Pedicle
d Vertebral artery
e C3

CT of neck with bone windows at level of hyoid and C3 vertebra, axial section

The hyoid bone has a body which curves in the midline and two greater horns which articulate laterally with the body. The stylohyoid ligaments attach to the lesser horns (not shown) of the hyoid. The hyoid lies at the C3 vertebral level.

A typical cervical vertebra is shown (C3). The major differences between cervical and other vertebrae are the inclusion of formina in the transverse processes and also the existence of anterior and posterior tubercles arising from the transverse processes. The transverse foramina allow transmission of the vertebral arteries to the skull; these are usually accompanied by veins and sympathetic nerves.

Q31 Answers

a Anterior arch of C1
b Lateral mass of C1
c Dens
d Posterior arch of C1 (neural arch)
e Transverse ligament of C1

CT of neck with bone windows at level of C1 vertebra, axial section

The first cervical vertebra is also known as the atlas as it 'holds up' the skull. The atlas is unusual by virtue of not having a vertebral body (the body has become detached from C1 and has fused with the body of C2 to form the dens); it is composed of two lateral masses and an anterior and a posterior arch. Note that the posterior arch is not considered to be composed of right and left lamina as in other vertebrae.

The dens is a superior projection of C2 which enables rotation of C1 on C2 (therefore termed the axis vertebra). The dens is held in place by a strong transverse ligament known as the transverse ligament of the atlas. This ligament is continuous with two vertical bands of connective tissue joining the occipital bone superiorly and the body of C2 inferiorly. Collectively these three ligaments form a cross over the posterior aspect of the dens known as the cruciform ligament.

Q32 Answers

a Anterior arch of C1 vertebra
b Nasopharynx
c Mylohyoid muscle
d Laryngopharynx
e Oesophagus

CT of neck with bone windows, midline sagittal section

The nasopharynx is the posterior extension of the nasal cavity and lies superior to the soft palate; it begins at the nasal chaonae which are the posterior openings of the nasal cavity. The oropharynx is continuous with the oral cavity and extends to the epiglottis. Inferior to the epiglottis, in continuity with and extending to the trachea is the laryngopharynx. The larynx contains the vocal cords.

The floor of the mouth is formed by the mylohyoid muscle which closes the inferior opening of the mandible and functionally acts to elevate the tongue, floor of mouth and hyoid when swallowing and speaking.

Q33 Answers

a Epiglottis
b Greater horn of hyoid bone
c Thyroid cartilage
d Cricothyroid membrane forming vocal cords
e Cartilaginous tracheal rings

CT scan through larynx shown with bone windows, coronal section

The larynx connects the pharynx with the trachea and contains the vocal cords. Several cartilaginous structures compose the larynx. The thyroid cartilage provides antero-lateral coverage of the vocal cords, while the epiglottic cartilage acts like a lid to cover the larynx when swallowing. The arytenoid cartilages sit on either side of the midline on the lamina of the cricoid cartilage. Attached to the anteriorly projecting vocal processes of the arytenoid are the vocal cords; movement here leads to changes in the length and tension of the vocal cords which is the means for vocalizing. The corniculate and cuneiform cartilages are very small structures attached to the arytenoid cartilage, these are not usually individually discernable with CT. The cricoid cartilage lies between the thyroid cartilage above and the trachea below and is the only complete ring of cartilage in the larynx or trachea.

Q34 Answers

a Right lobe of thyroid
b Sternocleidomastoid muscle
c Internal jugular vein
d Tracheal ring
e Isthmus of the thyroid

Ultrasound scan through right lobe of thyroid, axial section

The thyroid gland has two lobes which lie on either side of the trachea just inferior to the thyroid cartilage at the level of C5 to T1. These lobes are joined in the midline by an isthmus. The thyroid is enclosed within the pretracheal fascia and hence moves with the trachea during swallowing. Strap muscles (sternohyoid and sternothyroid) cover the thyroid and are visible in the image provided.

Immediately lateral to the thyroid lie the internal carotid arteries. Antero-lateral to these are the internal jugular veins. These major blood vessels to the head are protected throughout their superficial course within the neck by the sternocleidomastoid muscle.

The trachea is supported anteriorly by C-shaped arches of hyaline cartilage. These prevent the trachea from collapsing and are brightly echogenic on ultrasound.

Q35 Answers

a Pons
b Pituitary fossa containing the pituitary gland
c Skull base lines (McRae's line defines the opening of the foramen magnum) enable confirmation that cranial contents remain within the skull and also that there is not invagination of the dens of C2 from below.
d Superior medullary velum
e Epiglottis

T2W MRI, midline sagittal section

The pons is recognizable on midline sagittal section by its large anterior bulge ('pot belly'); this is composed of the cerebellopontine fibres which extend postero-laterally on either side to form the middle cerebellar peduncles.

The pituitary gland is a midline structure which rests within the bony sella turcica on the superior aspect of the sphenoid. On T1W weighted MR imaging the posterior lobe of the pituitary gland is normally high signal.

A thin layer of tissue extends between the superior cerebellar peduncles to form the roof of the 4th ventricle; this is known as the superior medullary velum.

Q36 Answers

a Parapharyngeal space
b Medial pterygoid muscle
c The facial nerve, external carotid artery and retromandibular vein pass through the parotid gland
d Internal carotid artery
e Masseter muscle

T1W MRI of neck at level of parotid glands, axial section

The parapharyngeal space is a triangular fatty filled area situated lateral to the pharynx and anterior to the major blood vessels for the head. It is important to recognize this area because it can be readily displaced and/or infiltrated by disease.

There are four muscles of mastication and these all attach to the mandible. Only the masseter muscle lies lateral to the mandible. The medial and lateral pterygoid muscles are so named because of their origin medial and lateral to the lateral pterygoid plate (an inferior process of the sphenoid bone). The medial pterygoid attaches distally to the medial aspect of the mandibular ramus, while the lateral pterygoid attaches to the neck of the mandible. The fourth muscle of mastication is the temporalis.

The parotid gland is the largest of the three paired salivary glands and sits between the ramus of the mandible and the mastoid process and extends down to the angle of the mandible with both a deep and a superficial lobe. The facial nerve

(CN VII) divides into its terminal branches within the parotid gland, therefore disease within the parotid can lead to ipsilateral facial palsy (lower motor neurone). The other major structures which can be seen passing through the parotid gland are the external carotid artery and the retromandibular vein (formed from the union of superficial temporal and maxillary veins).

Q37 Answers

a Hypoglossal nerve (CN XII)
b Epiglottis within oropharynx
c Vertebral artery
d Upper cervical spinal cord
e Sternocleidomastoid muscle

T1W MRI through neck at level of C2/3, axial section

Immediately posterior to the tongue is the oropharynx. This channel provides combined passage for both the foods we eat and the air we breathe. At rest the oropharynx is open to both the oesophagus and the trachea simultaneously. As a food bolus is propelled backwards by the muscular action of the tongue, the swallowing reflex is instigated. The hyoid bone rises in the midline bringing the epiglottis down over the laryngeal opening. Constriction of the pharyngeal muscles forces the food inferiorly where it is directed into the oesophagus.

Q38 Answers

a Sternocleidomastoid muscle
b Splenius muscle
c Trapezius muscle
d Spine of scapula
e Supraspinatus muscle

T1W MRI of posterior neck and shoulder muscles, coronal view

Each splenius muscle is composed of two parts (capitis and cervicis) which act as a single functional group. When both sides contract together they act to extend the head and neck. Independently, the splenius will perform lateral flexion and rotation of the neck to the same side. Lateral flexion also involves the ipsilateral sternocleidomastoid as well as other neck muscles.

The trapezius muscle covers the superior aspect of the shoulder and functionally is used to shrug the shoulders (upper fibres). The trapezius and sternocleidomastoid are innervated by the accessory nerve (motor, CN XI) and branches from the cervical plexus (sensory, C3/4).

Q39 Answers

a Sternocleidomastoid muscle
b Left lower anterior cervical nerve roots
c Scalene muscles
d Brachial plexus
e The brachial plexus nerve roots leave the root of the neck by passing between the anterior and medial scalene muscles

TIW MRI of neck showing brachial plexus nerve roots, coronal view

The brachial plexus provides nerve supply to the upper limb. It is formed from the anterior nerve roots of C5 to T1. These nerve roots pass between the anterior and medial scalene muscles to exit the root of the neck. The subclavian artery follows the same path between anterior and medial scalene muscles; the subclavian vein passes anterior to the scalenus anterior muscle. The scalene muscles also include scalenus posterior.

Q40 Answers

a Vertebral artery
b External carotid artery
c There are eight commonly described branches of the external carotid artery, these are: superior thyroid, ascending pharyngeal, lingual, facial, occipital, posterior auricular, superficial temporal and maxillary arteries
d Foramen lacerum within the petrous bone
e Aortic arch

Magnetic resonance angiography (MRA) of major head and neck arteries, anterior view

The major vessels supplying the head and neck are the paired common carotid and vertebral arteries.

The vertebral arteries arise from the subclavian arteries in the root of the neck. They course through the transverse formina of C6 to C1 vertebrae before entering the cranium via the foramen magnum to form the basilar artery in the midline. The vertebral arteries give off no branches in the neck.

The left common carotid artery arises directly from the aortic arch, while the right common carotid is one of the terminal branches of the brachiocephalic artery; the other is the right subclavian artery. At the level of C3/C4, both common carotid arteries bifurcate into their internal and external branches. The internal carotid begins postero-lateral to the external carotid artery. The internal carotid provides no branches within the neck, instead heading straight for the carotid canal in the skull base. Once through the carotid canal, the internal carotid artery turns 90 degrees antero-medially and passes through the foramen lacerum within the petrous temporal bone. Turning superiorly once again, the internal carotid enters the cavernous sinus within the cranial vault and undergoes two final turns before terminating as the anterior and middle cerebral arteries. The external carotid provides arterial blood to the upper neck, face (including scalp) and nasopharynx. There are eight commonly described branches of the external carotid artery (superior thyroid, ascending pharyngeal, lingual, facial, occipital, posterior auricular, superficial temporal and maxillary arteries), but individual variation is described.

2 THORAX

Q1

a Name the structure labelled A
b Name the structure labelled B
c Name the structure labelled C
d Name the structure labelled D
e Name the structure labelled E

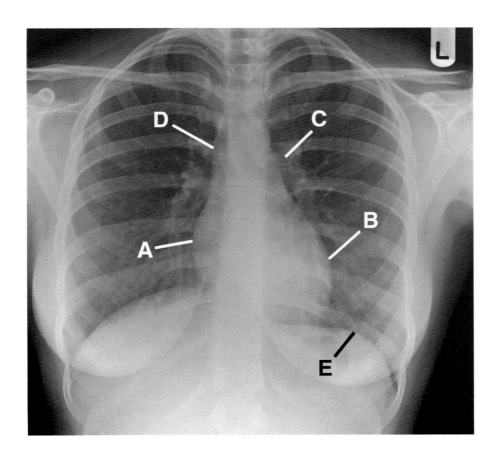

Q2

a Name the structure labelled A
b Name the structure labelled B
c Name the structure labelled C
d Name the structure labelled D
e Name the angle outlined and labelled E

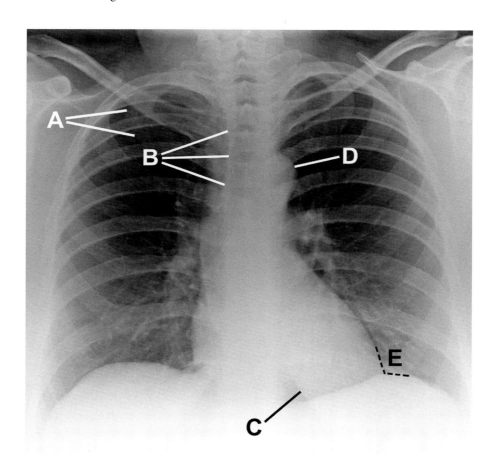

Q3

a Name the structure labelled A
b Name the structure labelled B
c Name the motor nerve supply of the structure labelled C
d Name the structure labelled D
e Name the structure labelled E

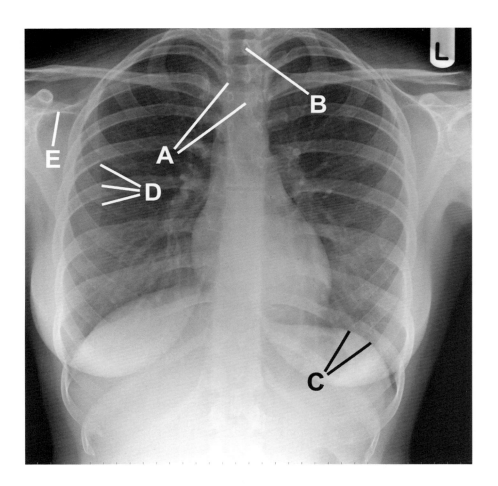

Q4

a Name the structure labelled A
b Name the structures located superior and inferior to the structure labelled A
c Name the airway labelled C
d Name the structure labelled D
e Name the anatomical variant demonstrated in this image

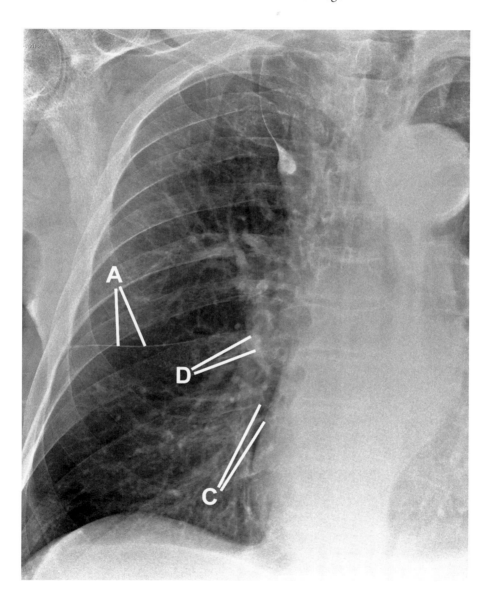

Q5

a Name the lymph node station indicated by label A
b Name the lymph node station indicated by label B
c Name the lymph node station outlined and indicated by label C
d Name the lymph node station indicated by label D
e Name the anatomical variant demonstrated on this image

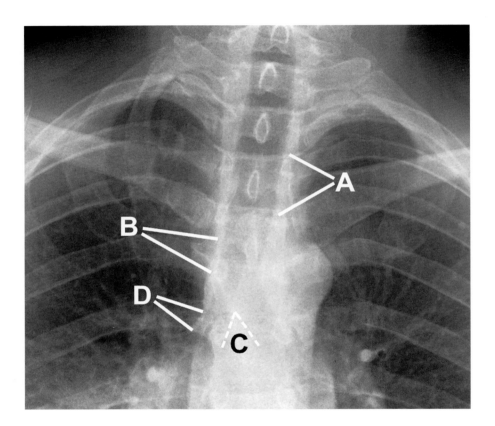

Q6

a Name the structure that lies in position A
b Name the structure that lies in position B
c Define the normal measurement of line C
d Name the structure labelled D
e Name the normal constituents of the structure outlined and labelled E

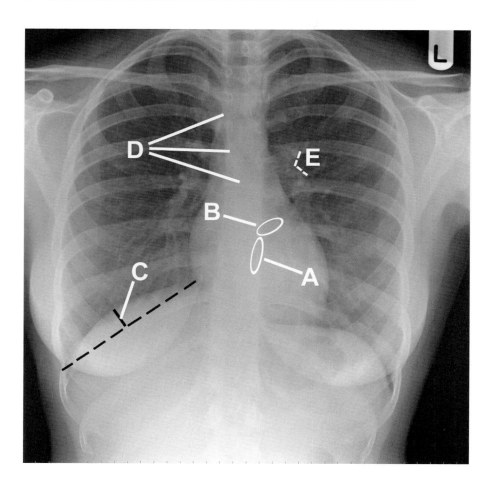

Q7

a Name the structure labelled A
b Name the structure labelled B
c Name the structures labelled C
d Name the structure labelled D
e Name the structure labelled E

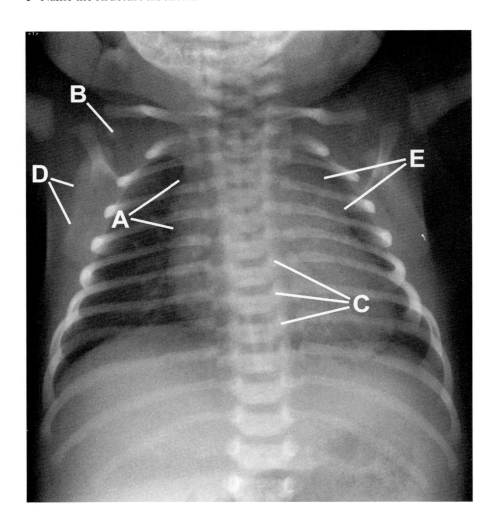

Q8

a Name the structure labelled A
b Name the structure labelled B
c Name the structure labelled C
d Name the structure labelled D
e Name the structure labelled E

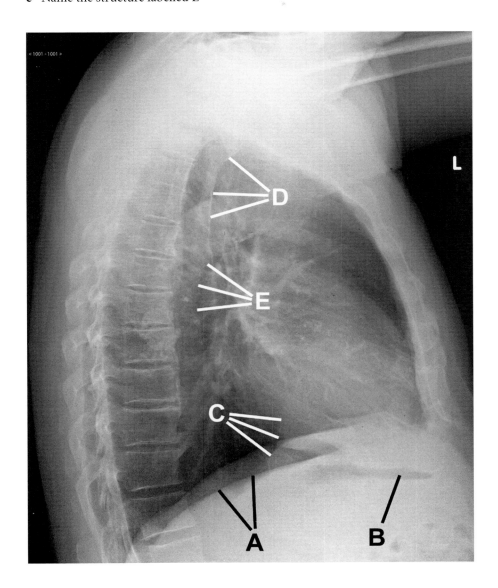

Q9

a Name the structure labelled A
b Name the structure labelled B
c Name the region outlined and labelled C
d Name the structure labelled D
e Name the structure labelled E

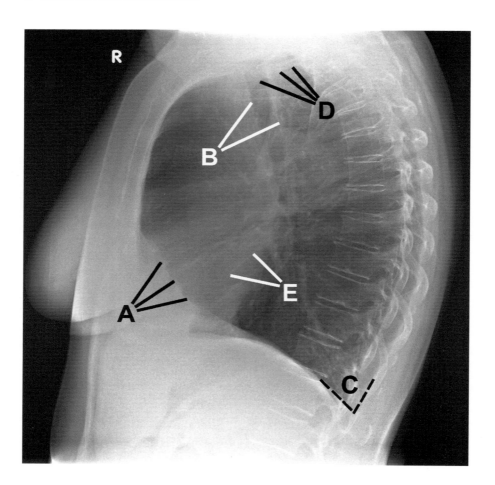

Q10

a   Name the structure labelled A
b   Name the joint space labelled B
c   Name the joint positioned lateral to B
d   Name the structure labelled D
e   Name the structure labelled E

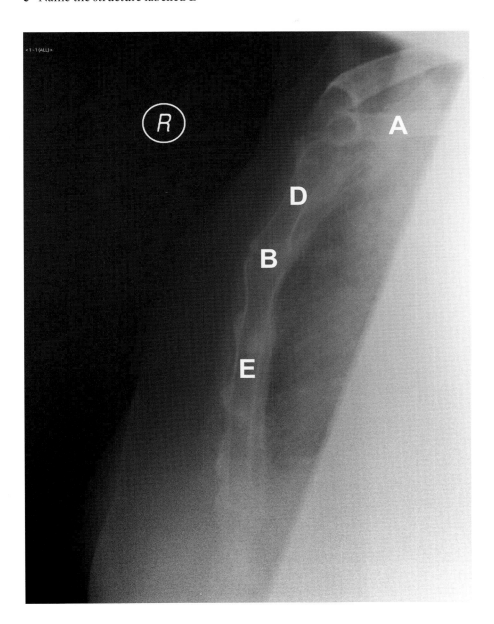

Q11

a Name the structure labelled A
b Name the structure labelled B
c Name the structures labelled C
d Name the tissue predominant in the area labelled D
e Name the type of structure labelled E

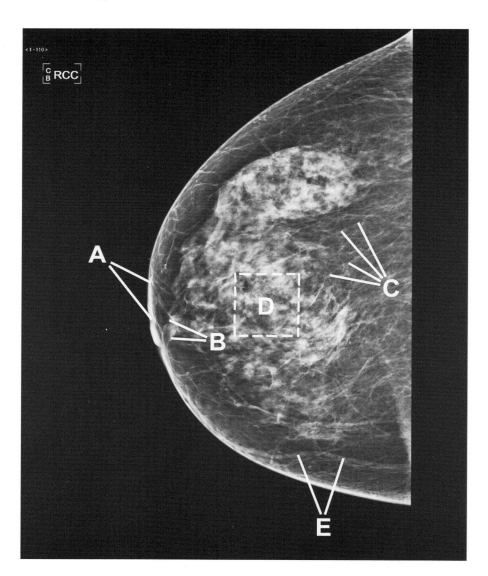

Q12

a Name the structure labelled A
b Name the structure labelled B
c Name the structure labelled C
d Name the structure labelled D
e Name the structure labelled E

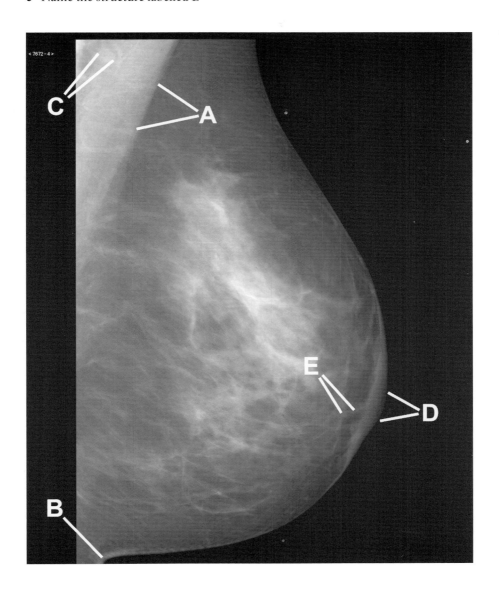

< 7672 - 4 >

Q13

a Name the structure labelled A
b Name the structure labelled B
c Name the structure labelled C
d Name the structure labelled D
e Name the structure labelled E

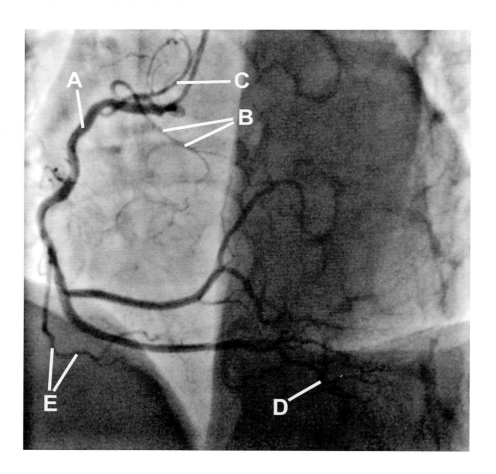

Q14

a Name the structure that creates the impression labelled A
b Name the structure that creates the impression labelled B
c Name the structure crossing the midline (right to left) posteriorly to the oesophagus at the level labelled C
d Name the linear structures labelled D
e Name the nodal group into which lymph from the oesophagus drains at position E

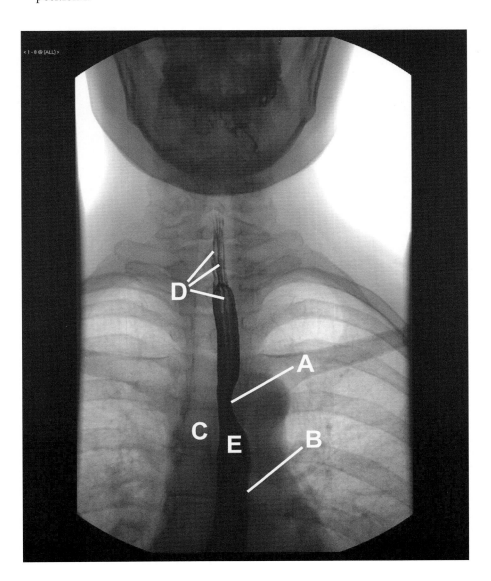

Q15

a Name the structure labelled A
b Name the parent artery whose branches supply the structure labelled A
c Name the vertebral level at the point labelled C
d Name the nerve(s) which crosses the diaphragm at the point labelled C
e Name the structure labelled E

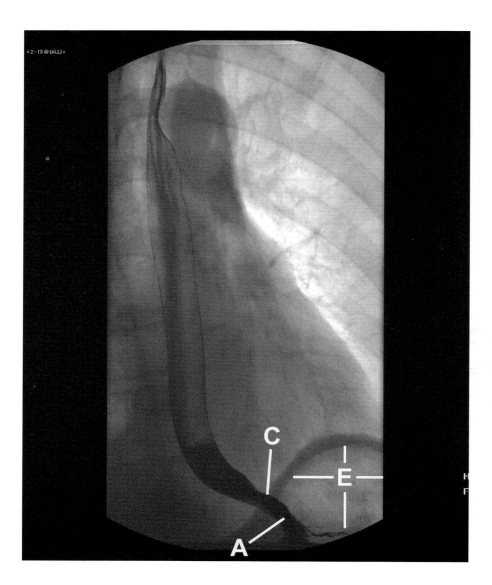

Q16

a Name the structure labelled A
b Name the structure labelled B
c Name the structure labelled C
d Name the structure labelled D
e Name the structure labelled E

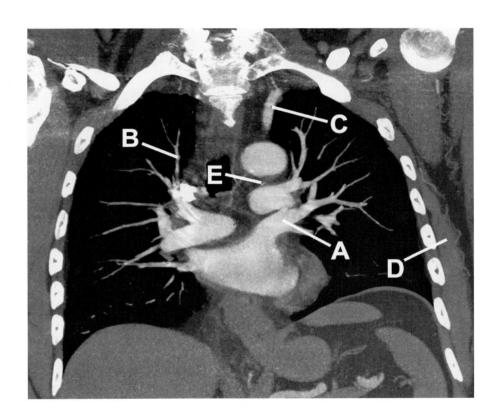

Q17

a Name the structure labelled A
b Define the upper limit of normal diameter of the structure labelled B
c Name the nerve located at the site labelled C
d Name the vertebral level of the corresponding diaphragmatic opening for the structure labelled D
e Name the additional structure(s) that cross the diaphragm through the same opening as structure D

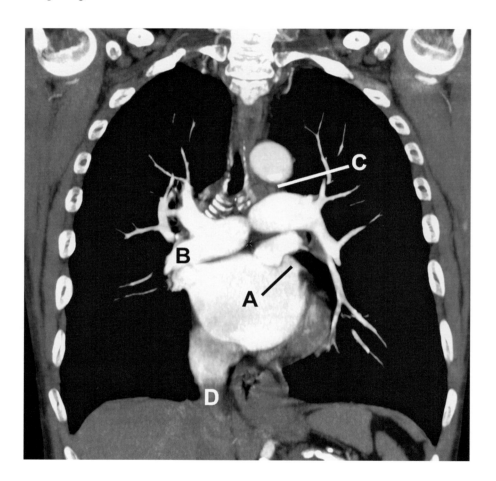

Q18

a Name the structure labelled A
b Name the structure labelled B
c Name the structure labelled C
d Name the structure labelled D (pointing at right carotid)
e Name the anatomical variant demonstrated in this image

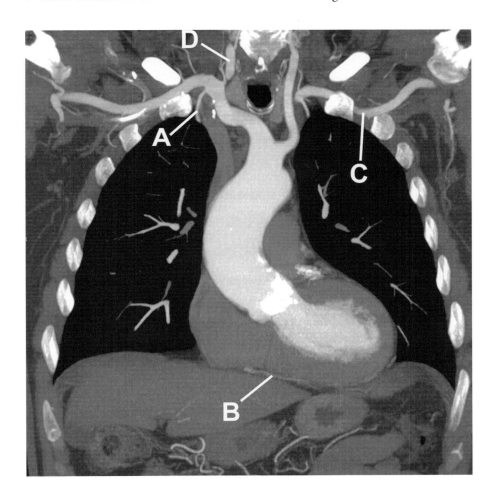

Q19

a Name the structure labelled A
b Name the structure labelled B
c Name the structure labelled C
d Name the structure labelled D
e Name the structure labelled E

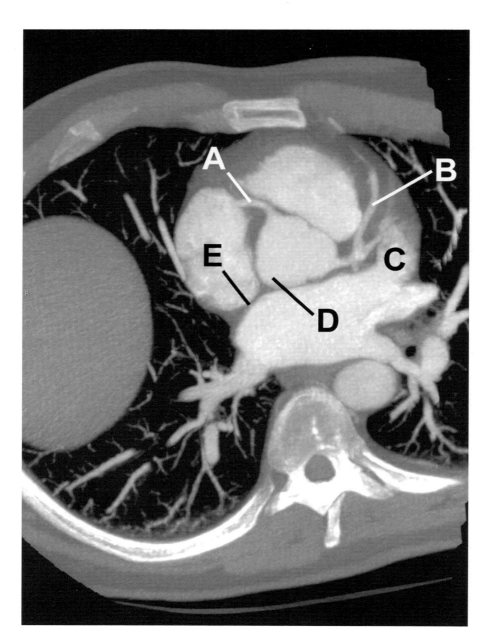

Q20

a Name the structure outlined and labelled A
b Name the structure labelled B
c Name the structure labelled C
d Name the structure labelled D
e Name the structure labelled E

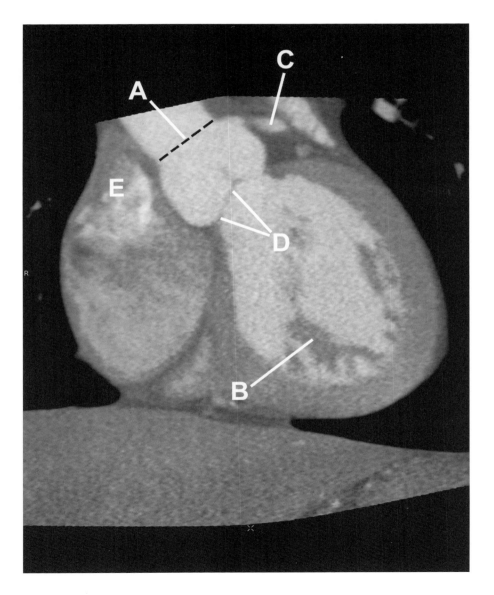

Q21

a Name the structure labelled A
b Name the structure labelled B
c Name the structure labelled C
d Name the structure labelled D
e Name the structure labelled E

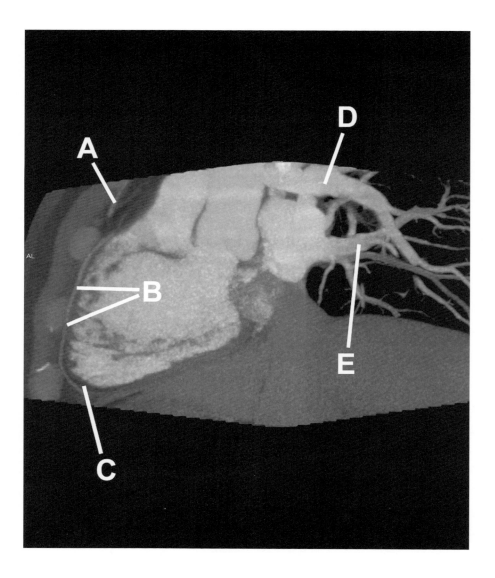

Q22

a Name the structure labelled A
b Name the structure labelled B
c Name the structure labelled C
d Name the structure labelled D
e Name the structure labelled E

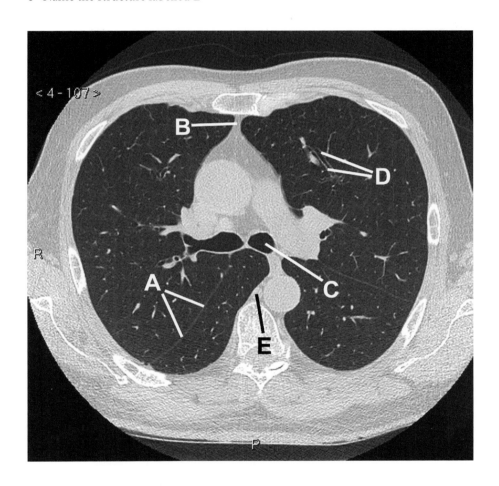

Q23

a Name the structure labelled A
b Name the structure labelled B
c Name the structure labelled C
d Name the structure that courses cranio-caudally anterior to the structure labelled C
e Name the structure that courses cranio-caudally posterior to the structure labelled C

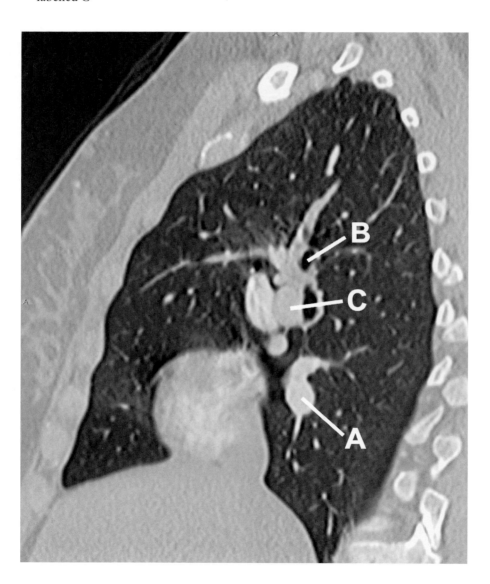

Q24

a Name the structure labelled A
b Name the structure labelled B
c Name the structure labelled C
d Name the muscle group labelled D
e Name the substance which is seen in greater abundance with increasing age at
   the site labelled E

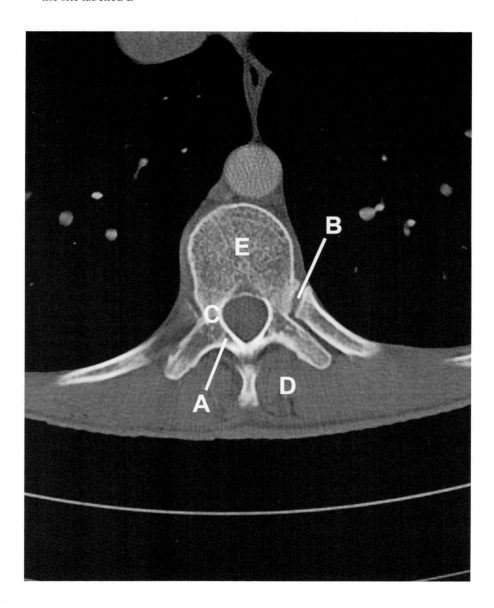

Q25

a Name the structure labelled A
b Name the structure labelled B
c Name the structure labelled C
d Name the structure labelled D
e Name the anatomical variant shown in this image

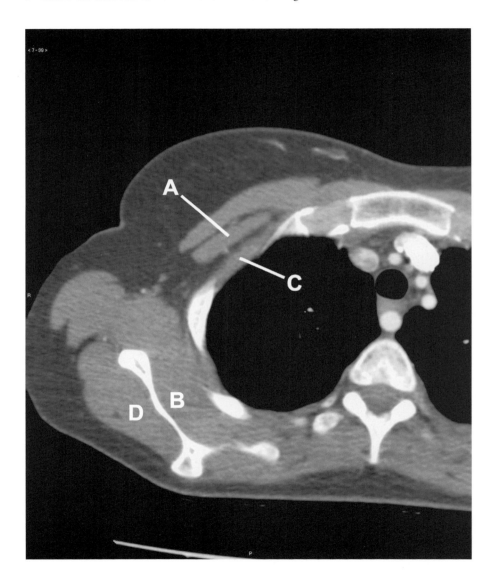

Q26

a Name the structure labelled A
b Name the structure labelled B
c Name the structure labelled C
d Name the structure labelled D
e Name the structure labelled E

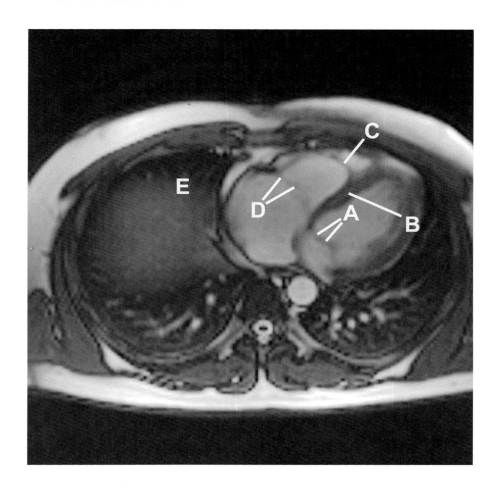

Q27

a Name the structure labelled A
b Name the motor nerve supplying the structure labelled B
c Name the structure labelled C
d Name the structure labelled D
e Name the structure labelled E

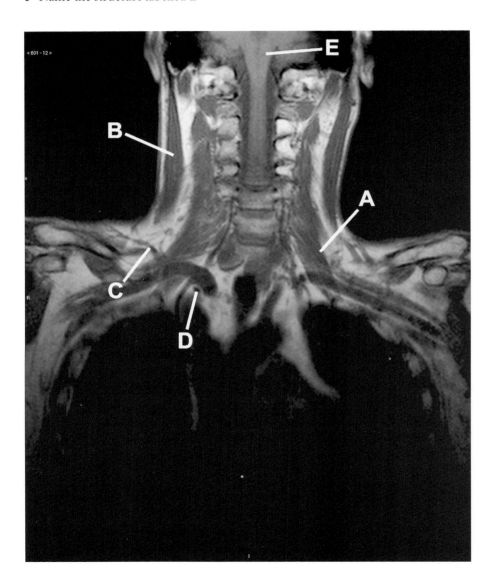

Q28

a Name the structure labelled A
b Name the structure labelled B
c Name the structure labelled C
d Name the structure labelled D
e Name the structure labelled E

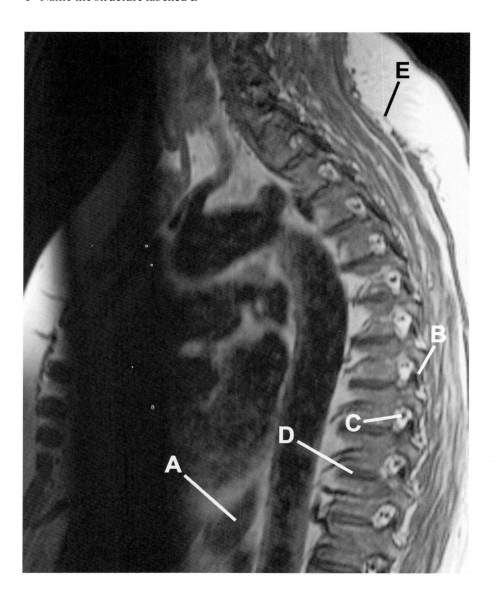

Q29

a Name the structures labelled A
b Name the structure labelled B
c Name the structure labelled C
d Name the insertion point(s) of the structure labelled C
e Name the structure labelled E

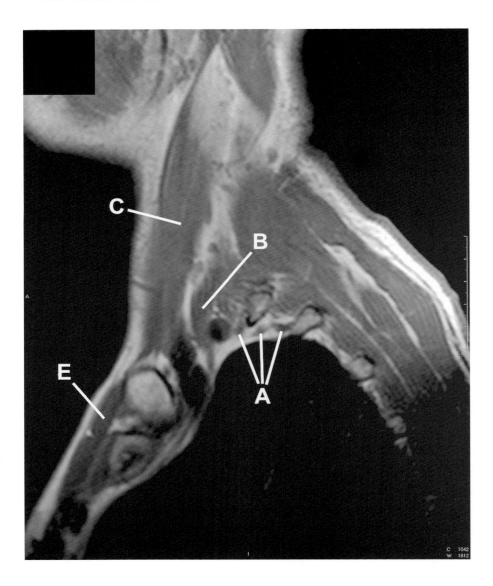

Q30

a Name the structure labelled A
b Name the structure labelled B
c Name the structure labelled C
d Name the structure labelled D
e Name the structure labelled E

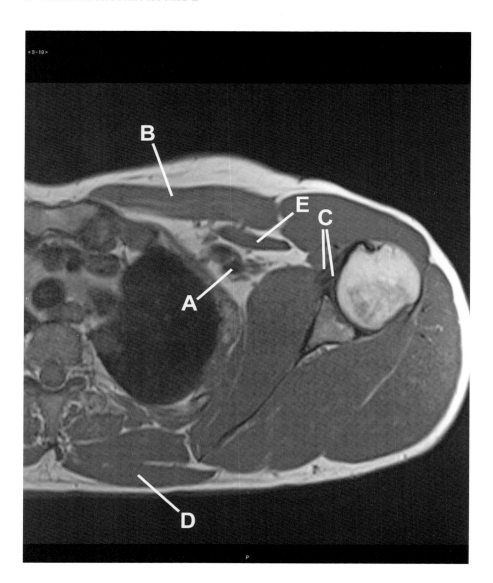

2

THORAX – ANSWERS

Q1 Answers

a Right atrium
b Left ventricle
c Left pulmonary artery
d Superior vena cava (SVC)
e Left hemi-diaphragm

Chest radiograph, PA projection

Cardiac and mediastinal silhouettes seen on the chest radiograph depend on there being contrast between the cardiac edge and adjacent aerated lung. Pathology within the chest can alter the appearance of one or more of these edges in a way that can enable accurate anatomical localization of the problem – the 'silhouette sign'.

The majority of the right cardiac border is made up of the right atrium with a small section of IVC inferiorly and the right hilum of the lung and SVC superiorly. From superior to inferior, the left mediastinal silhouette is formed by the left subclavian artery, distal aortic arch (aortic knuckle), pulmonary trunk and the hilum of the left lung. The left cardiac border is composed mostly of left ventricle, with the auricle of the left atrium forming the uppermost part of this border.

The left pulmonary artery spirals over the top of the left bronchus such that its branches come to lie posterior to the bronchi. The right pulmonary artery, longer than the left, passes anterior to the carina and at the lung root lies anterior to the bronchus. The right pulmonary artery gives off its branch to the upper lobe then enters the hilum where its branches also spiral over the bronchi to come to lie posterior to them.

Viewed from the front, the diaphragm curves up into the right and left domes. The highest point of the right dome is at the 6th intercostal space anteriorly (ranging from the 4th to the 7th). The left dome is usually 2cm lower than the right, although this may not be the case in all subjects. The level of the dome of the diaphragm can move about 4cm in deep respiration, but again there is a wide range of normal.

Felson B, Felson H. Localization of Intrathoracic Lesions by means of the Postero-anterior Roentgenogram: The Silhouette Sign. *Radiology* 1950; 55:363–374.

Q2 Answers

a Right 1st rib
b Paratracheal stripe
c Medial border of the left breast
d Aortic arch
e Left cardiophrenic angle

Chest radiograph, PA projection

The structures which create the mediastinal contour on a frontal radiograph are in part dependant on the age of the patient. The thymus is prominent in the superior mediastinum in paediatric patients and usually atrophies during childhood. The dense curved line on the right mediastinal border is formed by the ascending aorta, which lies relatively anterior in the chest. The distal aortic arch usually lies in the left posterior chest and is seen as the aortic knuckle.

The right paratracheal stripe is normally visible because the right upper pulmonary lobe lies immediately adjacent to the lateral tracheal wall. The opaque stripe is formed by the visceral and parietal pleura and some mediastinal fat. Normally the width should not exceed 3mm.

Breast shadows can produce lines which are projected over the chest.

Q3 Answers

a Trachea
b Spinous process
c Left phrenic nerve
d Medial border of right scapula
e Spine of right scapula

Chest radiograph, PA projection

The upper margin of the trachea as seen on a chest radiograph is approximately at the level of C6. It terminates at the carina, the position of which can vary depending on whether the radiograph is taken in inspiration (T4) or expiration (T6). The arch of the aorta and left-sided vessels lie along its left border and the pleura lies along the right (which forms the paratracheal stripe).

Vertebral spinous processes are viewed en face in this image.

Hemi-diaphragms are mainly innervated by the left and right phrenic nerves, which arise from spinal nerve roots C3–5 and supply all motor and most sensory innervation (sensory innervation of the peripheral diaphragm is partly through intercostal nerves). Phrenic neuropraxia or neuropathy results in the ipsilateral hemidiaphragmatic dome lying in a more cranial position than usual due to muscle relaxation. This can be idiopathic or as a result of mediastinal disease.

Scapular position in the frontal radiograph can vary. Asking the patient to put their hands on hips or overhead causes supero-lateral rotation of the scapula and therefore lessens the degree of overlay seen on the radiograph.

Naveed N. Good positioning is key to PA chest x-ray exams. 2001 www.auntminnies.com

Q4 Answers

a Horizontal (minor) fissure
b Anterior segment of upper lobe (superior) and the middle lobe (inferior)
c Bronchus intermedius
d Anterior segmental pulmonary artery
e Azygos fissure

Chest radiograph, AP projection

On a frontal radiograph, the visible line of the minor fissure consists of two layers of adjacent visceral pleura; the top layer from the anterior segment of the right upper lobe with pleura from the right middle lobe as the lower layer. On a frontal radiograph it runs transversely from the interlobar artery at the hilum, usually within 1cm of the hilar point, to the lateral aspect of the 6th rib.

Accessory fissures are occasionally present and the most common of these is the azygos fissure. As a result of incomplete migration of the embryological azygos vein through the right upper lobe, there remains a fissure of invaginated parietal and visceral pleura with the azygos vein lying at the base. This is seen on frontal radiograph as a curvilinear line running from the mediastinum through the right upper zone with a rounded opacity at its lower end. The section of right upper lobe between the fissure and mediastinum is termed the azygos lobe, however it is not an independent segment as it derives arterial and bronchial supply from the apical or posterior segment of the right upper lobe. A triangular area that marks the uppermost margin of the fissure is known as the trigone parietale. Stibbe (1919) classified the azygos lobe into being one of three types depending on the position of the trigone on the pulmonary apex. In type A, the trigone is located on the lateral aspect of the pulmonary apex; in type B, the trigone is situated in the midpoint of the cupula of the apex and in type C, the trigone is located on the medial aspect of the apex. Opacification of the normal azygos lobe has been described, especially in type B and C configurations.

On a frontal radiograph it is common to see one or both of the anterior segmental bronchi and arteries as rounded structures which are viewed 'end-on'. They should measure approximately 4–5mm diameter with the bronchus usually lying more laterally.

Stibbe EP. The Accessory Pulmonary Lobe of the Vena Azygos. *Journal of Anatomy* 1919; 53:305–314.

Caceres J. The Azygos Lobe: Normal Variants That May Simulate Disease. *European Journal of Radiology* 1998; 27:15–20.

Caceres J, Mata JM, Alegret X, Palmer J, Franquet T. Increased Density of the Azygos Lobe on Frontal Chest Radiographs Simulating Disease: CT Findings in Seven Patients. *Am J Roentgenol* 1993; 160:245–248.

Q5 Answers

a Left upper paratracheal nodes (2L)
b Right lower paratracheal nodes (4R)
c Sub-carinal nodes (7)
d Right tracheobronchial nodes (10R)
e Right cervical rib

Chest radiograph, PA projection, zoomed up view

Lymph nodes are located throughout the mediastinum and there is wide variation amongst normal individuals in their number and distribution. The descriptive nomenclature used does not correspond with the anatomical divisions of the mediastinum but is based on lymph node maps which have been variously defined by Naruke (1967) and Mountain (1996). A revised internationally standardized mapping criteria compiled by Rusch (2009) has been adopted by the American Joint Committee on Cancer (AJCC) and the Union Internationale Contre le Cancer (UICC).

The location of nodes are divided into numbered 'stations' with the suffix 'L' or 'R' to define laterality where needed. The boundaries of the stations are not symmetrical, reflecting differences in lymphatic drainage between the left and right lungs. There are 14 numbered stations in total.

In practical terms, when describing lymph nodes in the context of lung cancer staging there are three groups: ipsilateral hilar and/or tracheobronchial nodes (stations 10–14); ipsilateral mediastinal or sub carinal nodes (stations 1–9); and contralateral hilar or mediastinal, scalene or supraclavicular nodes. Involvement of these nodes defines N1, N2 and N3 disease respectively.

A cervical rib is the product of excessive elongation of the costal element of the seventh cervical vertebra. It may be an osseous or fibrous structure which extends to the first rib. These can cause compression of the subclavian artery and T1 nerve root at the thoracic outlet.

Naruke T. The spread of lung cancer and its relevance to surgery. *Nippon Kyobu Geka Gakkai Zasshi* 1967; 68:1607–1621.

Mountain CF, Dresler CM. Regional lymph node classification for lung cancer staging. *Chest* 1997; 111:1718–1723.

Rusch VW, Asamura H, Watanabe H *et al.* The IASLC Lung Cancer Staging Project: A Proposal for a New International Lymph Node Map in the Forthcoming Seventh Edition of the TNM Classification for Lung Cancer. *Journal of Thoracic Oncology* 2009; 4:568–577.

Sobin LH, Gospodarowicz MK, Wittekind C. *TNM Classification of Malignant Tumours,* Wiley-Blackwell, Chichester, 2009.

Edge SB, Byrd DR, Compton CC, Fritz AG. *AJCC Cancer Staging Manual,* 7th Ed, Springer, New York, 2010.

Q6 Answers

a Mitral valve
b Aortic valve
c >2.5cm
d Azygo-oesophageal stripe
e Superior pulmonary vein and lower lobe pulmonary artery (Hilar point)

Chest radiograph, PA projection

The cardiac valves are not usually visible on plain radiographs; however associated calcification or prosthetic implants can be seen. All four valves lie along a line from 3rd left to 6th right costal cartilages (or from the mid left atrium to the right cardiophrenic angle on chest x-ray (CXR)). In the frontal projection the mitral and aortic valves are positioned centrally. The mitral annulus is larger and usually orientated in a more vertical direction. The aortic valve is smaller and lies orientated at around 45 degrees to vertical. The lowest point of the aortic valve lies very close to the anterior annulus of the mitral valve and this is where the two are in fibrous anatomical continuity.

The diaphragmatic height can be calculated by drawing a line from the costophrenic angle to the cardiophrenic angle. Perpendicular measurement to the diaphragmatic dome should be >2.5cm, a height less than this suggests diaphragmatic flattening, possibly as a result of pulmonary hyperexpansion.

For descriptive purposes, when referring to pleural reflections around the mediastinum a 'line' typically measures <1mm in width, an example being the opposed layers of pleura of the fissures. A 'stripe' is typically >1mm wide and occurs when a mediastinal structure has gas on both sides (as in this case). An 'edge' is used to describe when structures of two different densities come into contact with each other.

The azygo-oesophageal stripe is formed where the azygos vein runs in close approximation to the right postero-lateral oesophageal margin. Following the course of the azygos vein, it is seen superiorly to veer towards the right. The right lung abuts the two structures at the azygo-oesophageal recess and, together with gas in the oesophageal lumen, forms this visible stripe.

The hilar point is formed where the superior pulmonary vein crosses the descending pulmonary artery. They should form an angle of approximately 120 degrees with the right hilar point projected over the 6th intercostal space and lying 1cm lower than the left.

Sussmann AR, Ko JP. Understanding chest radiographic anatomy with MDCT reformations. *Clinical Radiology* 2010; 65:155–166.

Q7 Answers

a Right lobe of thymus
b Secondary ossification centre of the coracoid process
c Pedicles of the vertebrae
d Lateral border of the scapula
e Left lobe of thymus

Chest radiograph in a neonate, AP projection

The major intra-thoracic anatomy of the newborn is largely similar to that of an adult with the notable exception of the thymus gland. The thymus is a lymphoid organ which is located within the anterior mediastinum; its relative volume is far greater in infants than in adults. On a frontal radiograph the thymus commonly creates an opacity extending from the mediastinum into one or both lung fields; however the classic description of a triangular 'sail' sign is not always seen. The normal thymus is not usually visible on a frontal radiograph beyond the age of five years.

Q8 Answers

a Left hemi-diaphragm
b Gas bubble in gastric fundus
c IVC
d Scapular spine
e Descending aorta

Right lateral chest radiograph

The dome of the left hemi-diaphragm is typically at a level inferior to that of the right and does not extend to the anterior chest wall due to the position of the heart. Along with the presence or absence of the gastric air bubble, these are features that can allow differentiation between the two hemi-diaphragms on a lateral chest radiograph.

The aortic arch can be seen in profile as it courses towards the back of the chest, becoming the descending aorta at around the level of the fourth thoracic vertebra. The superior and inferior vena cava both terminate at the right atrium and therefore lie towards the front of the chest (within the 'middle' mediastinum), with the IVC penetrating the right hemi-diaphragm at the level of T8 vertebral body.

To minimize composite bone overlap from the humerus, patients are asked to lift their arms out of the line of projection. This usually results in the scapula rotating externally and therefore entering into the field of view.

Padley S, MacDonald LS. *Grainger & Allison's Diagnostic Radiology*, Ch 12 – The Normal Chest, 5th Ed, Churchill Livingstone Elsevier, Edinburgh, 2008.

Ahmad N. Mastering AP and lateral positioning for chest x-ray. 2001 www.auntminnie.com

Q9 Answers

a Cardiac incisura (cardiac fat pad)
b Trachea
c Costophrenic recess (or sulcus)
d Left subclavian artery
e Oblique (major) fissure of left lung

Left lateral chest radiograph

The anterior aspect of the left lung base may come to lie in contact with the apex of the heart or more commonly with the epicardial fat pad. The latter of these will displace the lung from the antero-medial chest wall and can be mistaken for a mass lesion. The size and morphology of this fat pad can be variable, with rounded, angular and straight configurations described.

The costophrenic recess (or costophrenic sulcus) forms the inferior margin of the pleural cavity on both sides. Depth and location of the recess is dependant on, among other things, patient size, age and respiratory health. The lateral recess is seen readily on frontal radiographs, whereas the posterior aspect is best visualized using a lateral projection. On the right side, the posterior recess has been shown to be, on average, 3cm lower than the lateral costophrenic recess with its inferior aspect at the level of the L1 vertebral body.

Both the left subclavian and right brachiocephalic arteries travel postero-superiorly in the upper thorax and can be seen as they cross the air-filled trachea. The margin of the left subclavian artery can be seen to follow a gentle curve across the posterior aspect of the trachea. In contrast, the brachiocephalic artery has a slightly convex appearance in most people. The silhouette of both vessels should have only slightly curved margins and any striking linear convexity within this region could be the result of an underlying mass lesion.

Oh JK, Ahm MJ, Kim HL, Park SH, Shin E. Retrodiaphragmatic portion of the lung: how deep is the posterior costophrenic sulcus on posteroanterior chest radiography? *Clinical Radiology* 2009; 64:786–791.

Sussmann AR, Ko JP. Understanding chest radiographic anatomy with MDCT reformations. *Clinical Radiology* 2010; 65:155–166.

Q10 Answers

a Clavicle
b Manubriosternal joint
c 2nd sternocostal joint
d Manubrium
e Body of the sternum

Radiograph of the sternum, lateral view

The sternum is an anterior midline structure which gives structural support to the anterior thoracic wall. The upper bone is the manubrium. This has lateral articulations with the first costal cartilage by means of a primary cartilaginous joint. The manubriosternal joint is a symphysis where the manubrium articulates with the body of the sternum. This joint is slightly angulated (angle of Louis) and indicates the level of the 2nd sternocostal joint. Posteriorly the manubriosternal joint is at the level of the disc between vertebrae T4 and T5. Above this level is the superior mediastinum and below it the inferior mediastinum. The body of the sternum articulates with the costal cartilages of the 3rd–7th ribs by means of single synovial joints. At the inferior aspect of the sternum is the xiphisternal joint which is a symphysis between the body of the sternum and xiphoid process. The manubriosternal and xiphisternal joints frequently calcify in later life.

Q11 Answers

a Areola
b Retro-areolar duct
c Fibrous septae/suspensory ligaments of Cooper
d Fibro-glandular breast tissue
e Blood vessel

Mammogram left breast, cranio-caudal projection

The cranio-caudal projection is one of two views commonly used in breast radiography. Mammographic appearance of normal breast tissue depends on the proportion of fibro-glandular tissue to fat. It is usual for breasts to contain proportionally more fat with advancing age.

The skin of the areola is normally focally thickened. Retro-areolar ducts are seen as tubular densities which fan out into the breast from the nipple. Blood vessels within the breast can be very difficult to see and are only visible if surrounded by fatty tissue. Determining the type and location of a vessel is not always possible. Fine fibrous bands which run in a radial direction are another of the linear structures which are seen within the breast. These are the suspensory ligaments of Cooper which serve to support the structure of the breast.

Lymph nodes exist within the normal breast, especially within the upper outer quadrant. Normal nodes should be round or ovoid in shape, demonstrate a low soft tissue density and contain a fatty hilum.

Q12 Answers

a Pectoralis major muscle
b Infra-mammary skin fold
c Axillary lymph node
d Nipple
e Retro-areolar duct

Mammogram right breast, mediolateral oblique (MLO) projection

The MLO view of the breast demonstrates the pectoralis muscle, axilla and infra-mammary fold as well as the breast. The distribution and proportion of fibro-glandular breast tissue varies between patients and there is a wide range of 'normal' appearances. Wolfe (1976) described four categories of breast parenchymal distribution: N1, primarily fatty; P1, ≤25% prominent ducts; P2, >25% prominent ducts; and DY, dense fibroglandular tissue. Although not used in everyday clinical use, these categories can be used to ensure standardization when conducting research or audit.

Axillary lymph nodes are frequently seen on MLO mammograms. Although usually larger than those seen within the breast, the presence of fatty hilum remains useful in confirming their identity.

Wolfe JN. Breast patterns as an index of risk for developing breast cancer. *Am J Roentgenol* 1976; 126:1130–1137.

Q13 Answers

a Right coronary artery (RCA)
b Conus branch artery
c Sino-atrial node artery
d Posterior descending artery (PDA)
e Acute marginal branch artery

Right coronary angiogram, left anterior oblique (LAO)/cranial projection

Several angled projections are usually obtained to demonstrate all the parts of the tortuous coronary arteries. This example is a predominantly LAO projection with cranial angulation.

The conus branch supplies the right ventricular outflow tract. It arises as the first branch from the RCA (or occasionally from a separate small ostium in the right coronary sinus) in 60%. This artery arises from the circumflex in 40%.

The sino-atrial node artery is supplied in 60% from the RCA (the second branch). This heads posteriorly to supply the sino-atrial node, which is located in the superior aspect of the crista terminalis in the right atrium. In 40% this artery arises from the circumflex artery.

Branches given off by the mid-RCA supply the atria and ventricles including one or more acute marginal branches. In 85% the RCA terminates by becoming the PDA and one or more postero-lateral branches. At this point, there is usually a branch given off to the atrio-ventricular node.

'Dominance' in the coronary circulation is determined by the arterial system which supplies the PDA. In the example provided, the RCA gives rise to the PDA (right-dominant, the typical configuration). In 15% of individuals, either the circumflex artery supplies the PDA (left dominant) or there is combined supply of the PDA and postero-lateral arteries by the RCA and circumflex arteries respectively (co-dominant).

Libby P, Bonow RO, Zipes DP, Mann DL. *Braunwald's Heart Disease: A Textbook of Cardiovascular Medicine*, 8th Ed, Saunders, Philadelphia, 2007.

Lin EC *et al* . Coronary CT Angiography. 2010; eMedicine: www.emedicine.medscape.com

Q14 Answers

a Arch of the aorta
b Left main bronchus
c Thoracic duct
d Longitudinal mucosal folds of the oesophagus
e Posterior mediastinal nodes

Barium swallow examination, frontal view

Within the chest, normal impressions seen in the left wall of the oesophagus are (from superior to inferior) the aortic arch, left main bronchus and left atrium. A circumferential impression can often be seen at the level of the diaphragmatic hiatus. Aberrant vessels are a recognized cause of posterior impression (aberrant right subclavian artery) and anterior impression (aberrant left pulmonary artery).

The thoracic duct lies right and posterior to the lower thoracic oesophagus. It crosses the midline at the level of T5/6 then ascends along the left lateral aspect of the oesophagus behind the aorta and left subclavian artery. Drainage into the venous circulation occurs near the junction of the left internal jugular and subclavian veins.

Fine longitudinal folds are the typical mucosal appearance of the thoracic oesophagus.

Lymph from the upper oesophagus drains to the deep cervical nodes, the middle oesophagus drains to the posterior mediastinal nodes and the lower oesophagus to the para-aortic group of the coeliac nodes.

Q15 Answers

a Gastro-oesophageal junction
b Left gastric artery
c T10
d Left and right vagus nerves/vagal trunks (CN X)
e Air bubble in the gastric fundus

Double-contrast barium swallow, right anterior oblique (RAO) projection

The oesophagus courses forward and left in the lower chest where it passes in front of the aorta before crossing through the diaphragm hiatus at the level of T10. The hiatus is approximately 3cm left of the midline and the oesophageal wall often shows an indentation at this level. Crossing with the oesophagus through the diaphragm are the vagus nerves (CN X), branches of the left gastric vessels and lymphatics.

The oesophageal mucosa contains fine longitudinal folds measuring approximately 3mm thick whilst the gastric mucosal folds are seen to be thicker. The site of transition marks the gastro-oesophageal junction.

Arterial supply of the oesophagus can be divided into upper, middle and lower thirds. Branches of the inferior thyroid artery supply the upper; branches of the descending thoracic aorta supply the middle; and branches of the left gastric artery supply the lower third.

Q16 Answers

a Left superior pulmonary vein
b Right superior apical pulmonary artery
c Left subclavian artery (first part)
d Serratus anterior muscle
e Ligamentum arteriosum

CT pulmonary angiogram (CTPA), oblique coronal section

The pulmonary artery (PA) bifurcates soon after exiting the fibrous pericardium. The right PA is the longer branch and crosses the midline below the carina ending anterior to the right main bronchus at the hilum. Here it bifurcates into the right upper lobe branch and the interlobar branch, which supplies the middle and lower lobes. Thereafter pulmonary arteries are named in accordance with the segments supplied. Internationally standardized nomenclature of bronchopulmonary segmental anatomy was published by the British Thoracic Society in 1950 and can be seen below. Variations are common and there remains debate over what comprises a 'normal' configuration of segmental bronchopulmonary anatomy, as is described in the footnote.

Bronchopulmonary Segments:

RIGHT LUNG	LEFT LUNG
UPPER LOBE: apical, posterior, anterior	UPPER LOBE: apical, posterior, anterior, superior lingular, inferior lingular
MIDDLE LOBE: medial, lateral	
LOWER LOBE: apical (superior), anterior basal, lateral basal, posterior basal, medial basal	LOWER LOBE: apical (superior), anterior basal, lateral basal, posterior basal
TOTAL = 10	TOTAL = 9*

*Gray's Anatomy (40th Ed, 2008) and Applied Radiological Anatomy (2006) describe a combined apico-posterior segment of the left upper lobe. The latter text also does not list the medial basal segment of the left lower lobe as being a separate segment.

The shorter left pulmonary artery passes superior to the left main bronchus and runs within the concavity of the aortic arch. Here, the left PA and aorta are attached via the ligamentum arteriosum, the fibrous remnant of the foetal ductus arteriosus.

The subclavian artery arises on the left from the aortic arch, and on the right from the brachiocephalic artery (trunk). It is anatomically divided into three parts by the scalenus anterior muscle, to which the first part lies medially, second part lies posteriorly and third part lies laterally.

Pulmonary veins do not follow a segmental distribution, but travel in the intersegmental septae alongside lymphatic vessels. Usually two veins drain into each side of the left atrium, carrying blood from above and below the oblique fissures on both sides and entering the hilum slightly anterior to the PA. There are normal variations seen in the number of pulmonary veins (PV) draining into the atrium, for example three PV on the right or a single PV on the left.

Brock RC. The Nomenclature of Broncho-pulmonary Anatomy – An International Nomenclature Accepted by the Thoracic Society. *Thorax* 1950; 5:222–228.

Lee KS, Bae WK, Lee BH, Kim IY, Choi EW, Lee BH. Bronchovascular anatomy of the upper lobes: evaluation with thin section CT. *Radiology* 1991; 181:765–772.

Jardin M, Remy J. Segmental bronchovascular anatomy of the lower lobes: CT analysis. *Am J Roentgenol* 1986; 147:457–468.

Q17 Answers

a Left atrial appendage
b 2cm
c Left recurrent laryngeal nerve (branch of CN X)
d T8 (caval opening)
e Right phrenic nerve

CT pulmonary angiogram, coronal section

The left atrial appendage is a blind-ending recess positioned in the upper postero-lateral left atrium. This can be a site of mural thrombus formation, especially in patients with atrial fibrillation secondary to mitral valve disease.

The right interlobar artery can be seen on the PA chest radiograph running out lateral to the right cardiac border with bronchus intermedius in between. The diameter of the artery should not exceed 2cm (mean 1.4cm).

The recurrent laryngeal nerves supply the cervical trachea and oesophagus and the larynx. They are branches of the vagus (CN X) nerves which arise at the base of the neck on the right and down in the thorax on the left. On the right, the recurrent laryngeal nerve loops around the subclavian artery before heading cranially; on the left it passes under the arch of the aorta posterior to the ligamentum arteriosum, which runs between the aorta and left PA.

The caval opening in the diaphragm is at the level of the T8 vertebral body; the right phrenic nerve also crosses the diaphragm through this opening.

Bush A. Diagnosis of pulmonary hypertension from radiographic estimates of pulmonary arterial size. *Thorax* 1988; 43:127–131.

Q18 Answers

a Right internal mammary (internal thoracic) artery
b Posterior descending (interventricular) artery
c First part of the left axillary artery
d Right carotid artery
e 'Bovine arch'

CT aortic angiogram, maximum intensity projection, coronal section

The Bovine arch configuration of vessels shown in this image is the most common arch anomaly and is said to be present in 13% of the population. It is when the left common carotid artery arises from the right brachiocephalic trunk rather than the arch and results in there being only two arch branches. Despite its name, this arch vessel configuration is not the same as is found in cows and other ruminant animals. The actual 'bovine' aortic arch has a single large branch from which bilateral carotid and subclavian arteries arise. Despite this discrepancy, the term is widely used and understood in human medicine.

The first part of the subclavian artery is the section lying medial to scalenus anterior and gives rise to three branches. From proximal to distal these are the vertebral artery, thyrocervical trunk and internal mammary (or internal thoracic) artery. The last of these travels inferiorly in the chest wall alongside the lateral sternal edge.

Lateral to the first rib, the subclavian becomes the axillary artery. This is anatomically divided into three parts depending on the position relative to pectoralis minor, to which the first part is medial, the second part posterior and third part lateral.

Layton KF, Kallmes DF, Cloft HJ, Lindell IP, Cox CV. Bovine Aortic Arch Variant in Humans: Clarification of a Common Misnomer. *Am J Neuroradiol* 2006; 27:1541–1542.

Q19 Answers

a Right coronary artery (RCA)
b Left anterior descending (LAD) artery
c Left atrial appendage
d Non-coronary (or posterior coronary) sinus
e Interatrial septum

CT chest with intravenous contrast, maximum intensity projection, axial section

The right and left main coronary arteries originate from their respective coronary sinuses. The third sinus of Valsalva lies right posterior and is called the non-coronary sinus.

The RCA originates anteriorly and travels between the right auricle and infundibulum of the right ventricle. It then follows the atrio-ventricular groove down to the inferior cardiac margin giving off the sino-atrial (SA) nodal and conus branches. The nodal branch is variable in its origin arising from the RCA in 60% of individuals and from the left coronary artery (LCA), circumflex branch, in the remaining 40%. The posterior descending artery (PDA) travels along the base of the heart. In 85% of people, the RCA supplies the PDA in a 'right dominant system'.

The left main stem originates postero-laterally and travels between the left auricle and the pulmonary trunk. The circumflex continues on this same course, travelling over the left side of the heart along the atrio-ventricular groove. It gives off the obtuse marginal branches and in approximately 40% of people the sino-atrial (SA) nodal branch. The LAD courses along the interventricular groove on the anterior surface of the heart. It supplies diagonal branches to the left and right ventricles and also perforating branches to the interventricular septum.

The left atrial cavity is smooth-walled, indicating that it developed from the incorporation of the pulmonary veins into the wall of the developing heart. The roughened wall of the left auricle indicates that it is the remnant of what was once an embryological cardiac chamber. The atrio-ventricular (AV) node cannot be seen on diagnostic imaging; however its position is reasonably constant within the right atrium. It lies in the interatrial septum, above the insertion of the septal tricuspid valve leaflet and left of the opening to the coronary sinus.

Q20 Answers

a Sino-tubular junction
b Papillary muscle in the left ventricle
c Left main stem coronary artery
d Non-coronary (right posterior) aortic valve cusp
e Right atrial appendage (auricle)

CT coronary angiogram, coronal section

Distal to the aortic orifice the wall of the ascending aorta bulges into the three sinuses of Valsalva. The RCA originates from anterior (right coronary) sinus and the LCA from the left posterior (left coronary) sinus. They are positioned in accordance with the three cusps of the valve which allows for a wider opening and therefore reduction in the resistance of flow. Its transition to the ascending aorta is called the sino-tubular junction.

The atrioventricular valve cusps of both the tricuspid and bicuspid (mitral) valves are attached by means of chordae tendinae to papillary muscles. These arise from the wall of each ventricle and contract in systole pulling tightly on the valve leaflets and hence preventing retrograde flow. Rupture of a papillary muscle, a rare complication of myocardial infarction, results in an acute regurgitation through the mitral valve often leading to heart failure. In these cases, the postero-medial papillary muscle is twice as likely to be affected as the antero-medial papillary muscle. This is thought to be due to the postero-medial muscle being supplied by the LAD system alone while the antero-medial usually receiving blood supply from both the circumflex and LAD systems.

Above and to the left of the SVC opening is the right auricle, a large triangular muscular out-pouch of the right atrium. It sits adjacent to the aorta and the AV groove.

Minami H. Papillary muscle rupture following acute myocardial infarction. *Jpn J Thorac Cardiovasc Surg* 2004; 52(8):367–371.

Q21 Answers

a Left internal mammary (thoracic) artery
b Left anterior descending (LAD) artery
c Epicardial fat
d Right main pulmonary artery
e Right inferior pulmonary vein

Cardiac CT, maximum intensity projection, oblique section

This image demonstrates the close proximity of the LAD and left internal mammary artery. This is an oblique section taken approximately along the line of the interventricular septum/long cardiac axis.

The serous pericardium consists of two layers, the parietal and visceral pericardium. The visceral pericardium is attached to the surface of the heart whereas the parietal pericardium is attached to the inner aspect of the fibrous pericardium. The space between the visceral and parietal pericardia is the pericardial space or cavity which in health is little more than a potential space containing a few millilitres of lubricating pericardial fluid. These layers cannot normally be differentiated on CT. It is common to see a layer of epicardial fat in between the myocardium and the visceral pericardium.

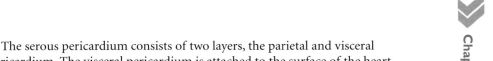
Q22 Answers

a Right oblique fissure
b Anterior pleural junction
c Left main bronchus
d Superior lingular segmental bronchus
e Azygos vein

High resolution CT chest, axial section

The oblique or major fissure separates the lower lobe from the remainder of the lung on both sides. The degree to which the fissures are developed is variable, with the transverse (horizontal) fissure being fully developed in only a third of people and absent in 10%. Underdevelopment can be difficult to determine radiologically. The line seen on plain radiographs is due to the composite layering of visceral pleura from both lobes surrounded by air and is only seen when viewing the fissure in profile (i.e. oblique fissure seen on lateral chest x-ray (CXR), transverse fissure seen on PA CXR). CT imaging normally displays the fissures as a clear line, but with underdevelopment of the fissure the position is indicated by a thin, dark linear strip which is devoid of traversing lung markings or vessels. The anterior junction of the pleura is responsible for the anterior junctional line that is seen on CXR and is the location of the sternopericardial ligaments.

Azygos means 'unpaired' and the azygos vein travels up the right paraspinal region, draining the posterior intercostal veins from the right side of the chest. It drains into the posterior aspect of the SVC, after having passed over the top of the right main bronchus. On the left are the hemiazygos (inferiorly) and accessory hemi-azygos (superiorly) veins. They provide drainage of the left inferior and superior posterior intercostal veins respectively and the two veins are occasionally in continuity. The hemiazygos veins usually cross the midline from left to right at the level of T9 to drain into the azygos vein.

Bronchi are named according to the lung segments which they supply. Juxta-cardiac lung is predominantly middle lobe on the right and lingula on the left. Both are divided into two segments with medial/lateral segments of the right middle lobe and superior/inferior segments of the lingula on the left.

Q23 Answers

a Inferior right pulmonary vein
b Right upper lobe bronchus
c Right pulmonary artery
d Right phrenic nerve
e Right vagus nerve

CT chest with intravenous (IV) contrast and lung windowing, sagittal section

The position of the pulmonary artery in relation to the bronchus can allow determination of whether it is right or left in the absence of other indicators. The right main bronchus is 'epi-arterial' (at the same level as the right pulmonary artery). The left main bronchus is 'hypo-arterial' (below the left pulmonary artery).

The superior pulmonary vein travels down through the hilum to reach the left atrium whilst the inferior vein approaches on a straighter course from the back.

The right main bronchus gives rise to the upper lobe branch soon after the carina and then continues as bronchus intermedius.

The vagus nerves pass posterior to the lung roots and cross the diaphragm alongside the oesophagus (vagal trunks). The phrenic nerves travel anterior to the lung root and down the antero-lateral surface of the pericardium to supply motor innervation to the diaphragm.

Q24 Answers

a Lamina
b Costovertebral joint
c Pedicle
d Erector spinae muscles
e Fat (yellow marrow)

CT thoracic spine, bone windows, axial section

The thoracic vertebrae are recognized in the axial plane by the presence of articulation with ribs. A synovial articulation occurs between the vertebral body and the head of the rib. Another articulation occurs between the tubercles of the rib and the anterior surface of the transverse process, known as the costotransverse joint. The vertebral bodies are slightly wedge-shaped in sagittal plane, which contributes to the kyphotic shape of the thoracic vertebral column. The pedicles pass back from the superior half of each vertebral body.

Extensor paraspinal muscles run the length of the spine lying in the vertebral grooves on either side of the spinous processes. The largest and most powerful of these is erector spinae, the component parts of which form the intermediate layer of the intrinsic back muscles.

In childhood the cancellous bone of the vertebral bodies contains red (haematopoetic) marrow, but this usually converts to yellow (fatty) marrow throughout adult life. At age 30 years, there will have been approximately 30% conversion and this continues over time. The appearance of vertebral bodies on MRI varies depending on the constituency of marrow. Red marrow shows greater contrast enhancement where as yellow marrow shows as higher signal on non-contrast T1W.

Q25 Answers

a Pectoralis minor
b Subscapularis
c Intercostal muscles
d Infraspinatus
e Aberrant right subclavian artery

CT upper chest with contrast, in arterial phase, axial section

The superficial muscles of the chest wall consist of pectoralis major and minor anteriorly; serratus anterior laterally; muscles of the shoulder girdle postero-laterally; trapezius and erector spinae posteriorly. The muscles which lie between the ribs (intercostals) are found in three layers: external, internal and innermost. The fibres of these muscles are orientated perpendicular to each other in a similar (though unrelated) fashion to the three muscles of the anterior abdominal wall. The intercostal neurovascular bundles run in the subcostal groove and are located between the internal and innermost muscle layers.

The four muscles that are principally responsible for stability and movement of the shoulder girdle are subscapularis, supraspinatus, infraspinatus and teres minor. Collectively they are known as the rotator cuff muscles.

An aberrant right subclavian artery takes its origin as the last branch from a left-sided aortic arch. It then crosses from left to right, passing behind the oesophagus in doing so. This can be a cause of posterior indentation seen in the oesophageal contour during barium swallow examinations and can occasionally be symptomatic (dysphagia lusoria).

Q26 Answers

a Mitral valve anterior leaflet
b Muscular interventricular septum
c Moderator band of the right ventricle
d Tricuspid valve anterior leaflet
e Right middle lobe of lung

Cardiac MRI, axial section

The atrioventricular valve cusps are tethered to the papillary muscles of the ventricular wall by chordae tendinae and act to prevent reflux of blood from the ventricle into the atrium. The bi-leaflet mitral valve is in the left heart; the anterior leaflet is the larger of the two and forms a division between the left ventricular inflow and outflow tracts. On the right side is the tricuspid valve, with leaflets sited in the anterior, posterior and septal positions.

The moderator band is a muscular bundle that crosses the right ventricular cavity, running from the lower interventricular septum to the anterior wall. It attaches at the level of the anterior papillary muscle and carries the right bundle branch fibres of the conducting system.

The interventricular septum is supplied via the septal branches of the left anterior descending (anterior interventricular) artery which runs the length of the anterior interventricular groove.

Q27 Answers

a Scalenus anterior muscle
b Right spinal accessory nerve (CN XI)
c Dorsal scapular artery
d Right recurrent laryngeal nerve
e Inferior cerebellar peduncle

T1W MRI base of neck, oblique coronal section

The scalenus anterior muscle and its relations are central to the anatomy of the root of the neck. It arises from the anterior tubercles of C3–6 in the form of four tendinous origins, passing infero-laterally and attaching to the upper surface of the first rib:

Anterior relations: Phrenic and vagus nerves (the right recurrent laryngeal branch loops beneath the 1st part of the right subclavian artery)
Ascending cervical, transverse cervical and suprascapular arteries
Internal jugular vein
Deep cervical lymph nodes

Medial relations: Inferior thyroid, vertebral, thyrocervical, internal mammary and subclavian (1st part) arteries
Vertebral veins
Ansa subclavia
Thoracic duct

Posterior relations: Costocervical, superior intercostal, deep cervical and subclavian (2nd part) arteries

Lateral relations: Dorsal scapular and subclavian (3rd part) arteries
Trunks of brachial plexus

The trapezius muscle is a large flat muscle which is the most superficial major muscle on the upper back. It arises posteriorly in the midline, from the skull to lower thorax, and converges to insert onto the inner aspect of the pectoral girdle at the clavicle, acromion and scapular spine. Motor nerve supply is from the spinal part of the accessory nerve which is the eleventh cranial nerve.

Q28 Answers

a Oesophagus
b Zygapophyseal (facet) joint
c Dorsal root ganglia within the intervertebral canal
d Intervertebral disc
e Ligamentum nuchae

T1W MRI cervical and thoracic spine, sagittal section

The distal oesophagus courses left and anterior, passing in front of the aorta before traversing the diaphragm at the T10 level.

Thoracic vertebral bodies articulate together through zygapophyseal (facet) joints. Positioned either side of the midline they are small synovial joints between the inferior articular processes of the vertebra above and the superior articular processes of the vertebra below. On the side of the vertebral bodies are costal demi-facets for articulation with the ribs. The first rib and lower two ribs have a slightly different configuration. T1 has a complete facet superiorly for articulation with the first rib, and a demi-facet inferiorly for articulation with the 2nd rib. Both T11 and T12 have only a single complete facet for articulation with their corresponding ribs.

Additional support to the vertebral column is given by the anterior and posterior longitudinal ligaments running anterior and posterior to the vertebral bodies and associated discs; the ligamentum flavum running between adjacent laminae; interspinous ligaments running between adjacent vertebral spinous processes and the supraspinous ligament (known as the ligamentum nuchae above C7) running along the tips of the spinous processes.

Intervertebral discs consist of a cartilaginous endplate, the annulus fibrosis and the nucleus pulposis. As a result of being firmly attached to the anterior longitudinal ligament the annulus has greater strength anteriorly. Degeneration of the nucleus pulposis results in dehydration which changes the MRI signal characteristics (darker on T2W images).

The intervertebral foramina lie between adjacent vertebrae with the pedicle of the vertebra above forming the roof and the pedicle of the vertebra below forming the floor. In the thoracic, lumbar and sacral regions they transmit the corresponding spinal nerve and its respective dorsal root ganglion as well as the smaller spinal artery and vein. (In the cervical region spinal nerves emerge above their corresponding vertebra with the 8th cervical spinal nerve emerging below the 7th cervical vertebra).

Q29 Answers

a The three trunks of the brachial plexus
b Scalenus anterior
c Sternocleidomastoid
d Manubrium and clavicle
e Pectoralis major

T1W MRI root of neck, sagittal section

The attachment of the scalenus anterior is onto the upper surface of the first rib. It passes between the subclavian artery and subclavian vein, with the artery lying deep to the muscle and running alongside the three cords of the brachial plexus. The anatomy of the brachial plexus is complex, and a full description is beyond the scope of this text. For simplicity it can be divided into sections which are (proximal to distal) the roots, trunks, divisions, cords and terminal branches. The roots refer to the anterior rami of the C5–T1 spinal nerve roots which come together to form three trunks in the neck. These divide into six divisions posterior to the clavicle (three anterior and three posterior) before reorganizing themselves again into three cords posterior to pectoralis minor. The cords surround the axillary artery and are named medial, lateral and posterior according to their position in relation to the artery as they enter the axilla before finally dividing into the terminal branches.

Sternocleidomastoid muscle arises from the mastoid process and occipital bone and passes obliquely downwards and forwards to insert medially into the manubrium ('sternal head') and clavicle ('clavicular head'). As an anatomical landmark, it forms the division of the anterior and posterior triangles of the lateral neck.

Q30 Answers

a Second part of Axillary artery
b Pectoralis major
c Tendon of subscapularis
d Trapezius
e Pectoralis minor

T1W MRI of upper chest and shoulder, axial section

The axillary artery is divided into three parts. The first part lies medial, the second part posterior and the third part lateral to pectoralis minor muscle. The axillary artery lies postero-lateral to the axillary vein.

As well as descriptively dividing the axillary artery into its three parts, pectoralis minor is the landmark used in delineating the three levels of axillary lymph nodes – level I are lateral to pectoralis minor, level II are posterior to pectoralis minor and level III are medial to pectoralis minor. The levels are utilized in the staging of breast cancer, for which nodal involvement is the single most important factor in determining prognosis. Involvement of level III nodes (N3a) carries a poorer prognosis than involvement of level I or II.

Singletary SE. Revision of the American Joint Committee on Cancer Staging System for Breast Cancer. *Journal of Clinical Oncology* 2002; 20:3628–3636.

Q1

a Name the structure labelled A
b Name the structure labelled B
c Name the structure that runs immediately lateral to the structure labelled B
d Name the structure labelled D
e Name the structures that connect the underside of the clavicle to the coracoid process

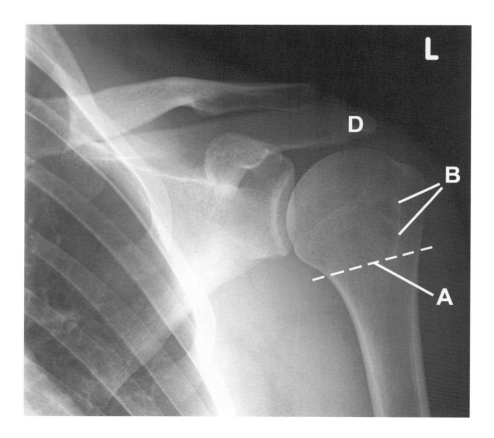

Q2

a Name the structure labelled A
b Name the structure labelled B
c Name the structure labelled C
d Name the structure labelled D
e Name the structure that lies at the centre of the 'Y' labelled as E

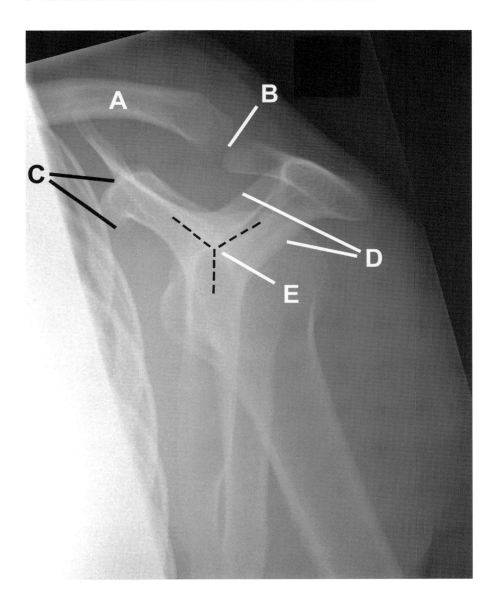

Q3

a Name the structure labelled A
b Name the structure labelled B
c Name the structure labelled C
d Name the structure labelled D
e Name the structure that runs through the groove labelled E

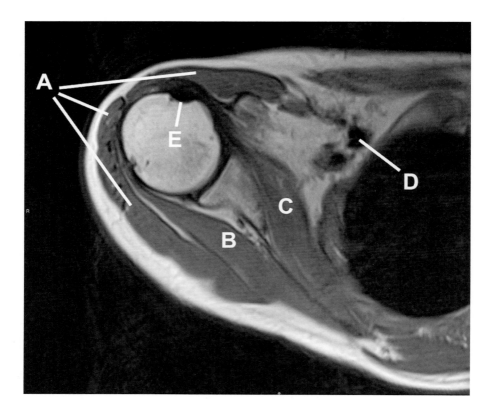

Q4

a Name the structure labelled A
b Name the high signalled structure labelled B
c Name the structure labelled C
d Name the structure labelled D
e Name the structure labelled E

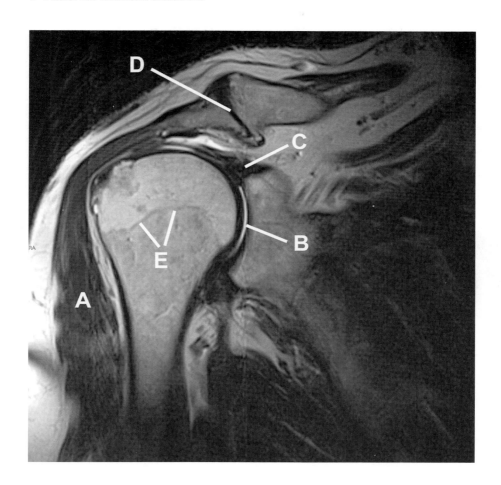

Q5

a Name the structure labelled A
b Name the structure labelled B
c Name the structure labelled C
d Name the structure labelled D
e Name the group of structures labelled E

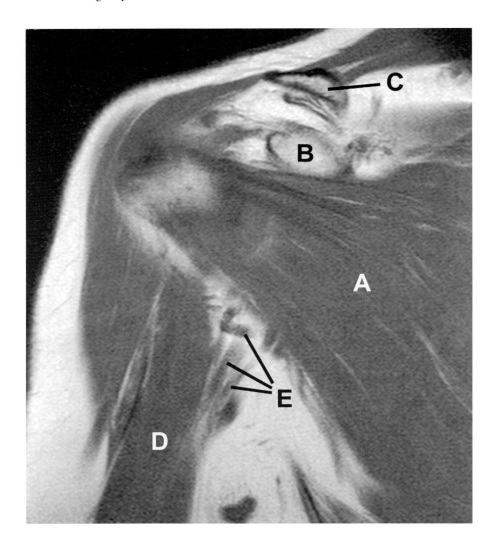

Q6

a Name the structure labelled A
b Name the structure labelled B
c Name the structure labelled C
d Name the structure labelled D
e Name the structure labelled E

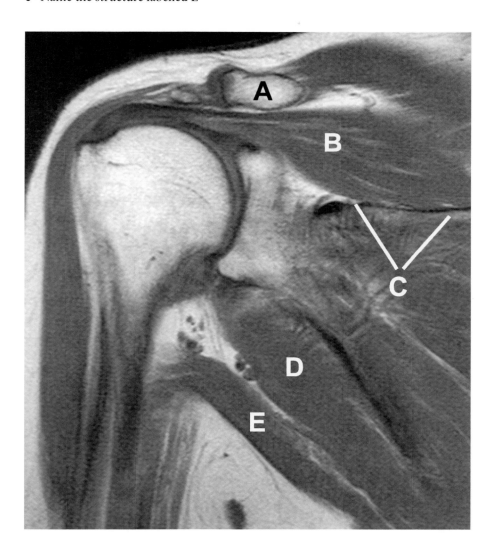

Q7

a Name the structure labelled A
b Name the structure labelled B
c Name the structure labelled C
d Name the structure labelled D
e Name the structure labelled E

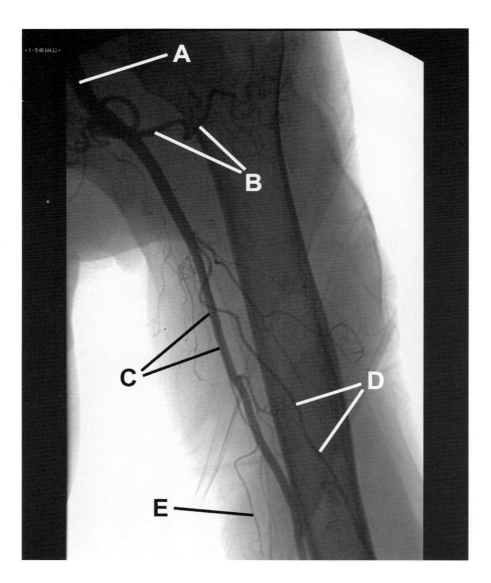

Q8

a Name the structure labelled A
b Name the structure labelled B
c Name the structure labelled C
d Name the structure labelled D
e Name the three major neurovascular structures found in the area labelled E

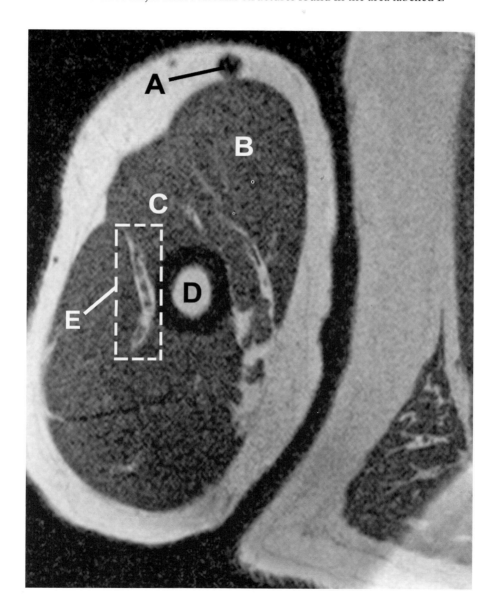

Q9

a Name the structure labelled A
b Name the vessels labelled B
c Name the vessel labelled C
d Name the structure labelled D
e Name the vessel labelled E

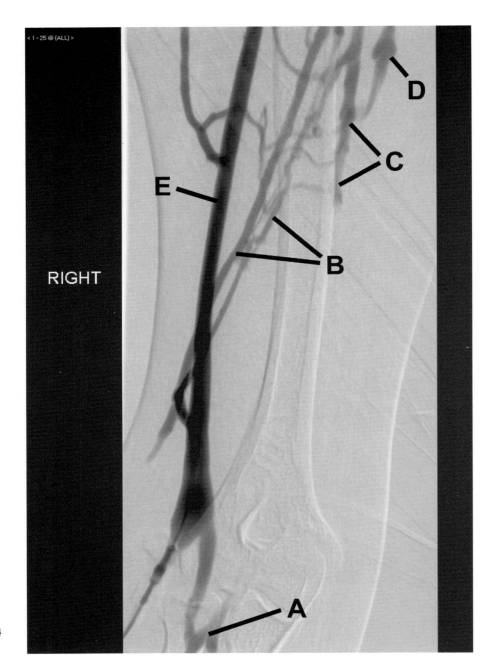

Q10

a Name the structure labelled A

b Name the soft tissue structure represented here in black and labelled B which allows rotation of the proximal radius on the neighbouring ulna

c Name the structure labelled C

d Name the flared part of the humerus labelled D

e Name the function of the major muscle group that attaches to E

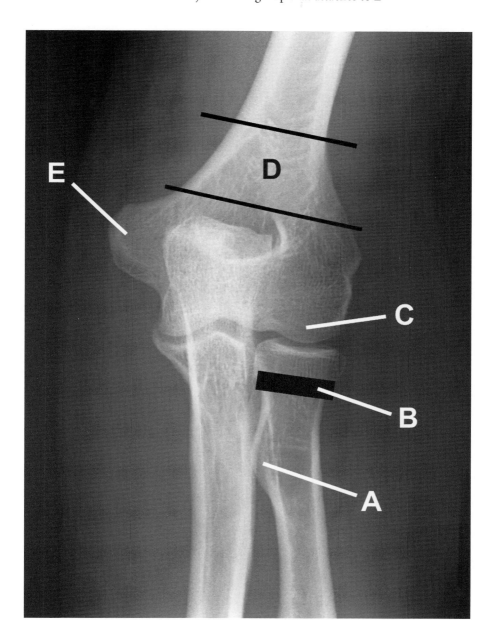

Q11

a Name the soft tissue structure labelled A
b Name the bony recess labelled B
c Name the line indicated by C
d Name the structure labelled D
e Name the structure labelled E

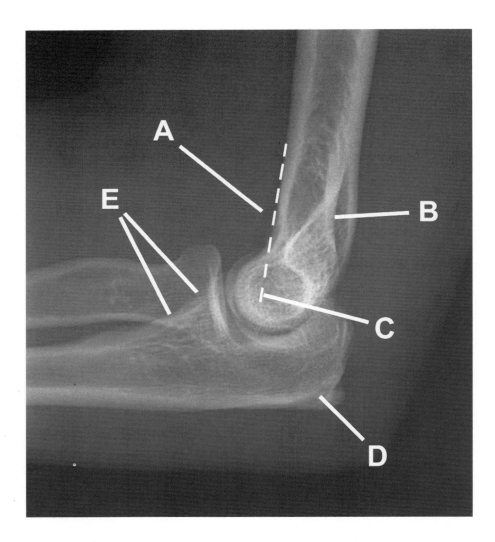

Q12

a   Name the structure labelled A
b   Name the structure labelled B
c   Name the structure labelled C
d   Name the structure labelled D
e   Name the structure labelled E

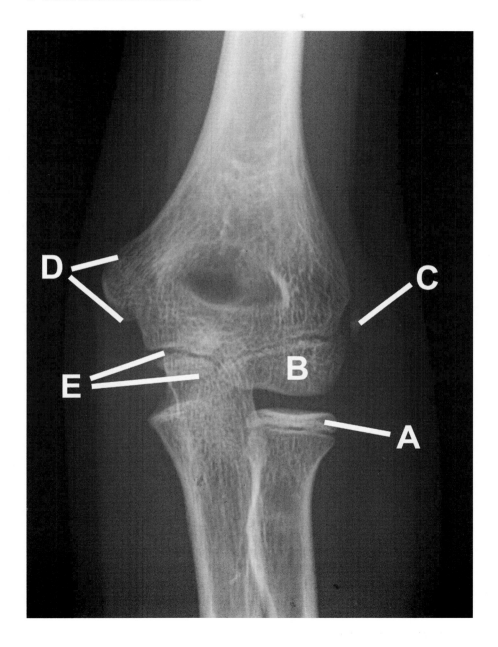

Q13

a Name the structure labelled A
b Name the structure labelled B
c Name the structure labelled C
d Name the structures labelled D
e Name the structures that B and C terminate as in the hand

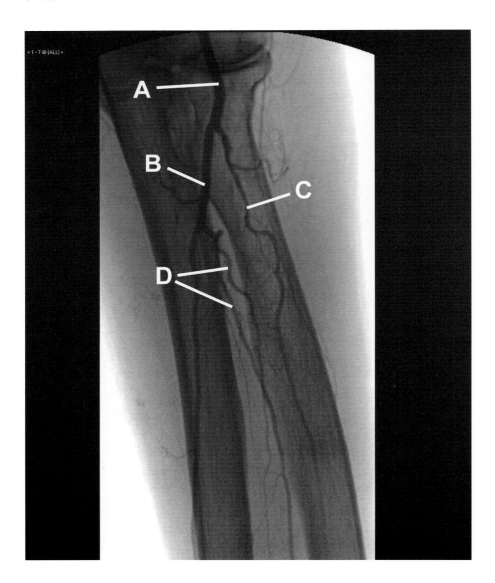

Q14

a Name the group of structures outlined and labelled A
b Name the structure labelled B
c Name the major function of the group of muscles labelled C
d Name the structure labelled D
e Name the structure labelled E

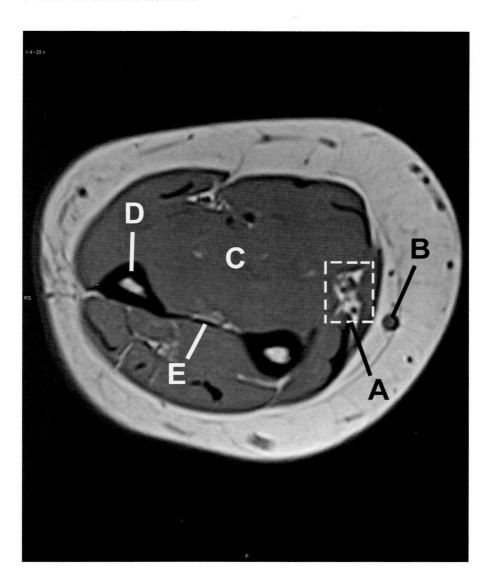

Q15

a Name the structure labelled A
b Name the structure labelled B
c Name the structure labelled C
d Name the structure labelled D
e Name the structure labelled E

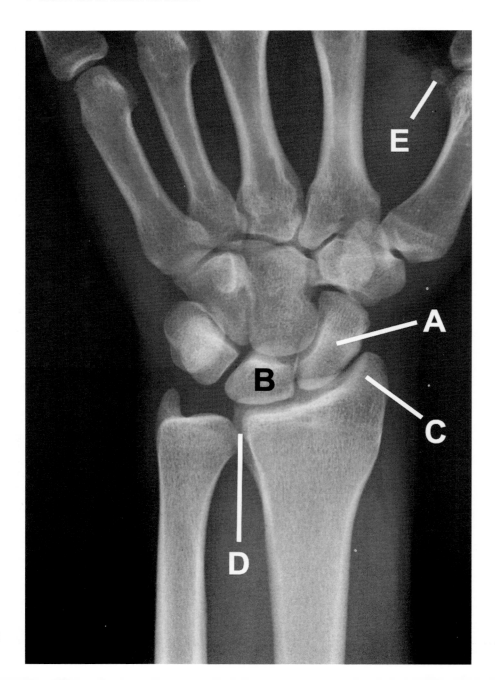

Q16

a Name the structure labelled A
b Name the soft tissue structure which articulates the distal ulna with the carpus and is located in the position labelled B
c Name the carpal bone labelled C
d Name the space indicated by D
e Name the carpal bone labelled E

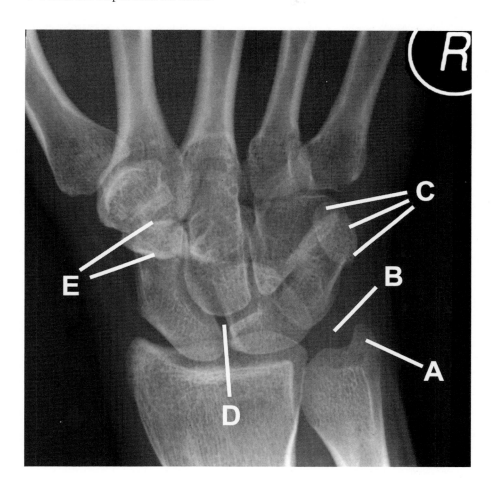

Q17

a Name the carpal bone labelled A
b Name the carpal bone labelled B
c Name the carpal bone labelled C
d Name the carpal bone labelled D
e Name the bone labelled E

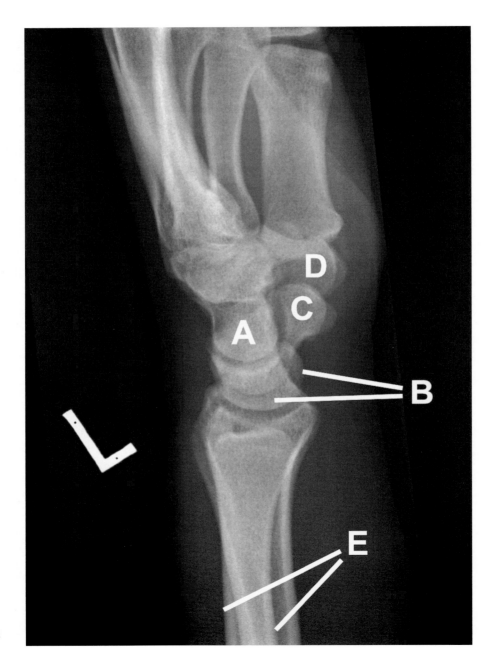

Q18

a Name the structure labelled A
b Name the three major structures outlined and labelled B
c Name the structure labelled C
d Name the major contents of the area labelled D
e Name the five carpal bones demonstrated

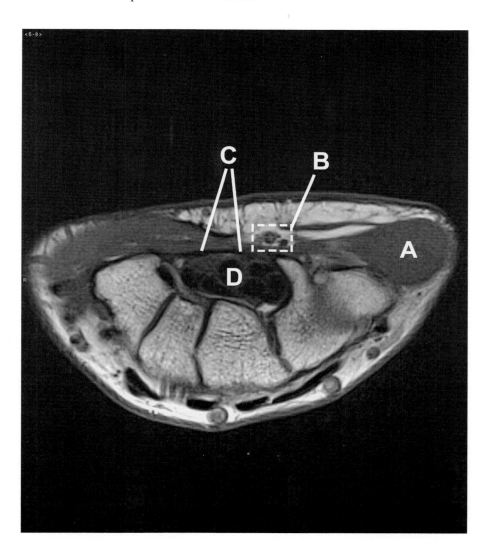

Q19

a Name the structure labelled A
b Name the structure labelled B
c Define the age by which ossification has begun in all eight of the carpal bones
d Name the structure labelled D
e Name the structure labelled E

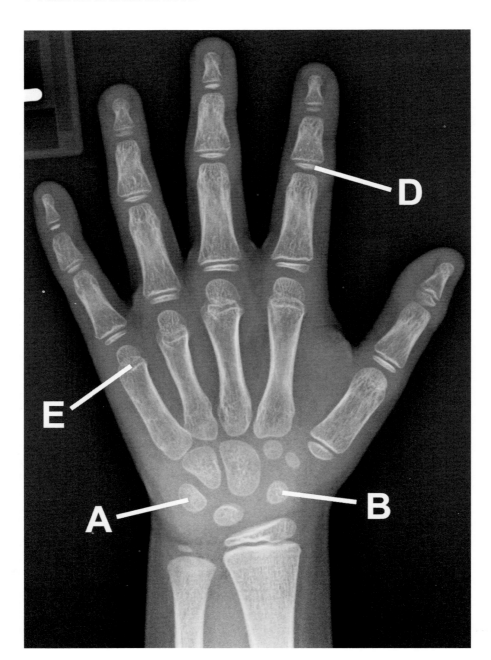

Q20

a Name the structure labelled A
b Name the structure labelled B
c Name the structure labelled C
d Name the structures labelled D
e Name the structure labelled E

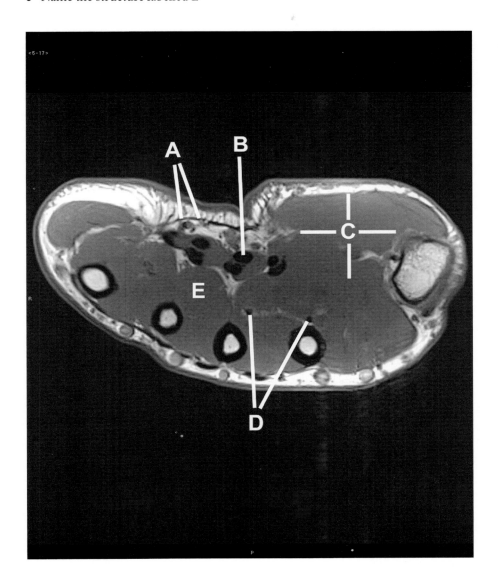

3

UPPER LIMB – ANSWERS

Q1 Answers

a Surgical neck of humerus
b Lesser tubercle of humerus
c Tendon of long head of biceps brachii
d Acromion process of scapula
e Trapezoid and conoid components of the coracoclavicular ligament

Radiograph of shoulder, AP view

The humerus has both anatomical and surgical necks. The anatomical neck defines the border of the articular surface which covers approximately half of the humeral head. The surgical neck is where the humeral head meets the shaft; fractures commonly occur at the surgical neck, hence the name.

Laterally, the humeral head has a greater and lesser tubercle. The tubercles are raised areas which allow for muscular attachment; the rotator cuff muscles attach to the tubercles of the humerus. Between the greater and lesser tubercles runs the inter-tubercular groove. The tendon of the long head of biceps runs through this groove before attaching to the superior lip of the glenoid within the joint capsule of the shoulder.

As well as the acromioclavicular joint (ACJ), the clavicle and scapula are linked via the coracoclavicular ligament which is made up of a laterally situated trapezoid ligament and the more medial conoid ligament. In cases of ACJ rupture the union between these two bones remains stable if the coracoclavicular ligaments are intact.

Q2 Answers

a Clavicle
b Acromio-clavicular joint space
c Coracoid process
d Spine of the scapula
e Glenoid cavity

Trans-scapular radiograph of the shoulder

The trans-scapular view of the shoulder is predominantly used to determine whether the humeral head articulates normally with the glenoid. The glenoid is identified as the point where the coracoid process, body and spine of the scapula meet; the humeral head should be projected centrally over this area. For further orientation, the coracoid process faces anteriorly (to the left of the image provided here).

Q3 Answers

a Deltoid muscle
b Infraspinatus muscle
c Subscapularis muscle
d Axillary vein
e The long head of biceps tendon runs through the inter-tubercular groove

T1W MRI of shoulder at level of gleno-humeral joint, axial view

The rotator cuff muscles of the shoulder comprise supraspinatus, infraspinatus, subscapularis and teres minor. The tendons of these muscles coalesce with the articular capsule of the shoulder joint and provide stability by holding the humeral head in place. Distally the rotator cuff muscles attach to the greater and lesser tubercles of the humerus, although only the subscapularis attaches to the lesser tubercle. All but the supraspinatus are rotators of the humerus (supraspinatus is active at the initiation of arm abduction).

The deltoid muscle forms the contour of the shoulder. Running from the outer aspect of the lateral third of clavicle, over the acromion and along the outer aspect of the spine of the scapula, it lies more superficially than the rotator musculature. The deltoid is the major abductor of the arm.

Proximally, biceps brachii has two attachments. The long head tendon runs through the intertubercular groove of the humerus to reach the supraglenoid tubercle of the scapula. The short head of biceps attaches to the coracoid process of the scapula.

Q4 Answers

a Deltoid muscle
b Trace of synovial fluid within gleno-humeral joint
c Superior glenoid labrum
d Acromio-clavicular joint
e Epiphyseal line (fused)

T2W MRI of shoulder, coronal view

The gleno-humeral articulation of the shoulder is a synovial ball and socket joint. It is normal to see a trace of synovial fluid with T2W MRI; in cases of joint disease or trauma this fluid volume may be significantly increased. The glenoid is naturally shallow providing only limited support for the humeral head. This support is enhanced by a circumferential fibro-cartilaginous ring known as the glenoid labrum. MRI provides a means of identifying and assessing the glenoid labrum which appears as a low signal triangular structure arising from the periphery of the osseous glenoid. Administration of contrast into the synovial joint space enhances visualisation of this area and will more reliably demonstrate a tear of the labrum.

Q5 Answers

a Subscapularis muscle
b Coracoid process of the scapula
c Distal end of clavicle
d Biceps brachii muscle
e Axillary neurovascular bundle

T1W MRI of shoulder, coronal section

It can be difficult with a single cross sectional image to orientate oneself with the anatomy. Coronal sections of the shoulder are usually aligned with the scapula which lies at an oblique angle (approximately 30 degrees antero-medially to postero-laterally) to the shoulder in the true coronal plane. The pectoralis major can be confused with the subscapularis in this scenario. Note however the region of muscle attachment; the subscapularis attaches to the lesser tubercle of the humerus which is part of the humeral head. Conversely, the pectoralis major attaches along the lateral edge of the intertubercular groove more distally on the humerus near the surgical neck. The MRI section provided here is anterior to the humerus but posterior to the thorax on the anterior border of the scapula. It is worth looking at an axial view of the shoulder on MRI to appreciate the orientation of this view. Note also the trapezius and deltoid muscles in this image.

The axillary neurovascular bundle runs anterior to the subscapularis muscle as it enters the arm.

Q6 Answers

a Acromion process of the scapula
b Supraspinatus muscle
c Spine of scapula
d Teres minor muscle
e Teres major muscle

T1W MRI of shoulder, coronal section

The four rotator cuff muscles of the shoulder are the supraspinatus, infraspinatus, teres minor and subscapularis. The supraspinatus tendon runs through the subacromial space (as shown) where it is prone to 'wear and tear', especially if there is bony stenosis of the space.

The teres major muscle lies nearly parallel with the teres minor and also originates from the lower border of the scapula. The teres major is different in its distal attachment; it is not part of the rotator cuff, instead it attaches to the medial lip of the intertubercular groove more distally on the humerus.

The axillary nerve (a posterior branch of the brachial plexus supplying deltoid and skin over deltoid) and circumflex humeral vessels pass through the space between teres major and minor (as shown). This is known as the quadrangular space; its medial and lateral borders are the long head of triceps and the humerus, respectively.

Q7 Answers

a Axillary artery
b Circumflex humeral artery
c Brachial artery
d Deep brachial artery (profunda brachii)
e Superior ulnar collateral artery

Fluoroscopic angiogram of the arm, AP view

Arterial blood to the upper limb is predominantly supplied by the axillary artery; numerous anastomoses exist around the scapula which can provide collateral supply in the event of axillary artery obstruction. At the lower border of the axilla (inferior border of teres major) the axillary artery becomes the brachial artery. The final branches of the axillary artery are the posterior and anterior circumflex humeral vessels; these arteries anastomose in a circle around the surgical neck of humerus. The brachial artery runs down the medial aspect of the arm and ends in the antecubital fossa where it bifurcates to form the radial and ulnar arteries. In addition to supplying the arm with arterial blood, several collateral vessels are derived from the brachial artery from different points along its course. These collaterals regroup around the elbow providing alternative blood supply to the forearm. The most notable include the deep brachial artery which follows the course of the radial nerve posteriorly behind the humerus and also the superior and inferior ulnar collateral arteries.

Q8 Answers

a Cephalic vein
b Biceps brachii muscle
c Brachialis muscle
d Medullary cavity of the humerus
e Radial nerve, deep brachial artery(s), deep brachial vein(s)

T1W MRI arm, axial section proximal to the midpoint of humerus

Venous drainage of the arm has superficial and deep components. The major superficial veins are the basilic and cephalic; the cephalic runs anteriorly over the arm while the basilic follows a more medial path. The deeps veins are named after their accompanying arteries.

The biceps brachii and brachialis muscles are the forearm flexors; the biceps brachii also acts to supinate the forearm. The arm is divided into anterior and posterior muscle compartments; collectively, biceps brachii and brachialis compose the anterior compartment of the arm. The three heads of the triceps brachii muscle form the posterior muscular compartment. These compartments are separated by medial and lateral intermuscular septi.

The radial nerve runs laterally through the arm posterior to the humerus in the plane between anterior and posterior muscular compartments. The deep brachial artery and vein follow the same course as the radial nerve through the arm at this level.

Q9 Answers

a Confluence of the radial and ulnar veins/origin of the brachial vein
b Deep brachial veins
c Brachial vein
d Venous valve
e Cephalic vein

Fluoroscopic venogram right arm, AP view

Venous drainage of the upper limb is divided into deep and superficial components.

The superficial veins are numerous and for the most part variable in their position. The cephalic and basilic veins are the major superficial veins of the arm and are more consistent in their path; they originate from a venous plexus on the dorsum of the hand and then travel up the medial (basilic) and lateral (cephalic) aspects of the arm. The superficial veins drain into the deep system via numerous perforating veins. Ultimately the basilic vein drains into the brachial vein in the upper arm while the cephalic vein drains more proximally into the axillary vein.

The deep veins of the arm are paired with the arteries both in name and with respect to the course they take.

Veins are recognizable on fluoroscopy by the existence of valves. These are periodically situated along the vessels and can be recognized as a short dilated segment; often the valve leaflets are seen within this segment (see image, labelled D).

Q10 Answers

a Radial tuberosity
b Annular ligament
c Capitulum
d Metaphysis
e Flexor muscles of the forearm

Radiograph of a skeletally mature elbow, AP view

The tendon for biceps brachii attaches to the radial tuberosity. There is also a bicipital aponeurosis which attaches more medially to the fascia of the forearm.

The annular ligament forms a collar around the head of the radius allowing radial rotation, a movement performed during pronation and supination of the forearm. Knowledge of the annular ligament is important as the radial head can be subluxed from this attachment in cases of 'pulled elbow' in children.

The capitulum of the humerus articulates with the radial head (the prefix *capit* indicates head).

The flared part of any long bone adjacent to the epiphyseal plate is known as the metaphysis.

Forearm flexors attach to the medial epicondyle (the common flexor origin – the site of pain in 'golfers elbow') while forearm extensors attach to the lateral epicondyle (the common extensor origin – the site of pain in 'tennis elbow').

Q11 Answers

a Anterior fat pad
b Olecranon fossa
c Anterior humeral line
d Olecranon process
e Coronoid process of ulna

Radiograph of a skeletally mature elbow, lateral view

The anterior fat pad (intracapsular, extrasynovial) is normally visible on a true lateral radiograph of the elbow. There is also a posterior elbow fat pad which normally resides in the olecranon fossa and is therefore not usually visible. An elbow effusion of any cause can raise the posterior fat pad out of the olecranon fossa making it visible on a lateral radiograph, i.e. the *posterior fat pad sign*.

The olecranon fossa is a recess on the posterior aspect of the distal humerus which allows space for the olecranon process of the ulna when the elbow is fully extended.

If a line is drawn down the anterior aspect of the humerus on a lateral elbow view, this line should bisect the anterior third of the trochlea. Supracondylar fractures of the humerus can disrupt this normal alignment.

Q12 Answers

a Epiphysis of radial head
b Epiphysis of capitulum
c Epiphysis of lateral epicondyle
d Epiphysis of medial epicondyle
e Epiphysis of trochlea

Radiograph of elbow in a 12 year-old child, AP view

Skeletal development at the elbow involves six epiphyses. These growth centres ossify in a consistent order although the age for the appearance of each centre can vary between individuals. It is important to remember the order in which these growth centres appear on plain radiography so that all bony fragments can be accounted for and none are missed. The medial and lateral epicondylar epiphyses in particular, are prone to injury and can appear in abnormal positions following trauma. The order in which these bony growth centres appear is remembered by the acronym CRITOE: The capitulum (C) appears first, usually around one year of age. Next is the radial head (R), and then the medial or internal (I) epicondyle; these are seen around five years of age. The trochlea (T) is seen around 11 years, closely followed by the olecranon (O) at 12 years. Finally, the lateral or external (E) epicondyle is usually apparent by 13 years of age.

Q13 Answers

a Brachial artery
b Ulnar artery
c Radial artery
d Anterior and posterior interosseous arteries
e Superficial and deep palmar arches

Fluoroscopic angiogram of forearm, AP view

The brachial artery traverses the antecubital fossa to reach the upper forearm before dividing into its two terminal branches at the level of the radial neck. The radial artery runs laterally while the ulnar artery runs medially through the forearm. Just distal to its origin, the ulnar artery gives off the common interosseous artery which quickly divides into the anterior and posterior interosseous arteries. These arteries are so named because they travel along either side of the interosseous membrane which connects the adjacent internal surfaces of the bony radius and ulna. In the hand, the radial and ulnar arteries both contribute to anastomotic connections in the form of the superficial and deep palmar arches. By this means, the entire hand can potentially be supplied by either of these two major arteries.

Q14 Answers

a Radial neurovascular bundle (radial artery, nerve and vein)
b Cephalic vein
c Flexion and of the wrist and fingers
d Ulna
e Interosseous membrane

T1W MRI of mid forearm, axial section

There are three major neurovascular bundles in the forearm; radial, median and ulnar. In addition there are anterior and posterior interosseous bundles; these lie on either side of the interosseous membrane. The radius appears more rounded in cross section when compared with the ulna.

The superficial veins are numerous in the forearm and are found in the subcutaneous fat which is superficial to the deep fascia (the deep fascia covers the muscular compartments). The cephalic and basilic veins are two of the most recognizable superficial veins; the cephalic runs on the lateral side of the arm, while the basilic runs medially. These vessels are continuous throughout most of the arm; they arise from a common plexus of superficial veins on the dorsum of the hand and are joined within the antecubital fossa by the median cubital vein.

Two major muscle groups are functional in the forearm. The flexors lie anterior and as a group are bulkier than the posteriorly situated extensor compartment of muscles.

Q15 Answers

a Scaphoid
b Lunate
c Radial styloid process
d Distal radioulnar joint
e Sesamoid bone on the thumb

Radiograph of the distal forearm and wrist, AP view

The eight carpal bones lie in two rows of four. The proximal row contains, from lateral to medial, the scaphoid, lunate, triquetrum and pisiform. With the exception of the pisiform these bones form a semicircle, the convexity of which is proximal and articulates with the corresponding concave surface of the radius. The distal row is formed, again from lateral to medial, by the trapezium, trapezoid, capitate and hamate; these bones articulate with the proximal row at the mid-carpal joint. The bones within each row articulate at intercarpal joints.

The ulnar surface of the distal radius has a notch for articulation with the ulna – the distal radioulnar joint. Holding the radius and ulna together at the distal radioulnar joint is the triangular cartilage running from the medial surface of the radius to the styloid process of the ulna. Situated laterally is the pyramidal radial styloid process.

In the thumb, a pair of sesamoid bones articulate with the flexor surface of the metacarpal head. They are contained within the tendons of flexor pollicis brevis and adductor pollicis.

Q16 Answers

a Ulna styloid
b Triangular fibrocartilage
c Pisiform
d Scapho-lunate joint space
e Trapezoid

Radiograph of right carpus, oblique view

The distal ulna appears shorter than the adjacent radius at the wrist on plain radiographs. What is not apparent on these images is the existence of the triangular fibrocartilage; this intracapsular structure articulates with the distal ulna and with the triquetral and lunate carpal bones. The triangular fibrocartilage can be visualized on MRI and arthrography can better demonstrate its integrity; if disrupted, intracapsular contrast can spill into the distal radio-ulnar joint.

With an AP view of the wrist, the scaphoid and lunate normally overlap slightly. On this oblique view the joint space is however, visible.

Q17 Answers

a Capitate
b Lunate
c Scaphoid
d Trapezium
e Ulna

Radiograph of wrist, lateral view

When viewed laterally, the lunate normally rests within the cup-shaped distal end of the radius. Similarly, the capitate sits within the distal hollow formed by the curve of the lunate; i.e. capitate sits within lunate sits within radius. This configuration is disrupted in lunate and perilunate dislocations which are best demonstrated with the lateral view. The other carpal bones are more difficult to recognize when viewed laterally as there is too much overlap, however by remembering that *the trapezium sits under the thumb*, this bone can also be identified. Due to differences in the appearance of their styloid processes, the radius and ulna can also usually be differentiated.

Q18 Answers

a Hypothenar eminence
b Ulnar nerve, ulnar artery and vein
c Flexor retinaculum
d Median nerve, four flexor digitorum superficialis tendons, four flexor digitorum profundus tendons and the tendon for flexor pollicus longus
e Trapezium, trapezoid, capitate, hamate, pisiform (as seen left to right of the image)

T1W MRI of wrist at level of carpal tunnel, axial section

The flexor retinaculum forms the roof of the carpal tunnel and extends from the hook of hamate and pisiform medially to the tubercles of the trapezium and scaphoid laterally. The major contents of the carpal tunnel are the median nerve, the four flexor digitorum superficialis tendons, the four flexor digitorum profundus tendons and the tendon of flexor pollicus longus. The flexor retinaculum can be surgically divided as treatment for carpal tunnel syndrome where there is compressive median nerve neuropathy. Note that the ulnar nerve does not travel through the carpal tunnel and is spared in cases of carpal tunnel syndrome.

There are two muscular prominences on the palmar surface of the hand; the thenar and hypothenar eminences. These muscle groups are responsible for flexion, abduction and opposition of the thumb and little finger (5th digit), respectively.

Q19 Answers

a Triquetral
b Scaphoid
c 12 years
d Epiphysis for the middle phalynx of the index finger
e Physis for the 5th metacarpal

Radiograph of the hand and wrist in a 7 year-old child, AP view

There are multiple ossification centres in the developing hand and wrist. The carpal bones ossify in a predictable fashion; the capitate and hamate are visible by one year of age, the triquetral by two years, the lunate by three years, the scaphoid, trapezoid and trapezium appear by six years of age while the pisiform is expected by the age of 12 years. A child's physiological age can be estimated by comparing the extent of bony development against published radiographic standards of normal. In such calculations, the epiphyses of the metacarpals and digits are often assessed, it is therefore important to know where each epiphysis belongs in relation to its parent bone. The metacarpal epiphyses lie distal to the bone (this can be confused with or mask a common injury to the 5th metacarpal), while the phalangeal epiphyses lie proximally.

Q20 Answers

a Palmar aponeurosis
b Tendon of flexor digitorum superficialis for the middle finger
c Thenar eminence
d Palmar digital arteries
e Lumbrical muscle to ring finger

T1W MRI of hand, axial section through midpoint of metacarpals

The palmar aponeurosis is a thickening of the deep fascia within the palm; it supports and protects structures in the palm.

The median and ulnar nerves terminate in the palm with branches supplying both muscles and skin of the hand. Similarly, the deep and superficial arterial palmar arches give off branches to the hand and fingers; each finger receives blood from a single common palmar digital artery that further divides into medial and lateral proper digital branches. These digital branches run the length of the finger.

Finger flexion is achieved through the action of several muscles. The long flexors of the fingers are the flexors digitorum superficialis (FDS) and profundus (FDP). There are four tendons for each (one to each finger) with the profundi lying deep to the supericialis throughout their course. For each of the four digits, the tendon of FDS splits and is attached to the sides of the middle phalynx. Through this split passes the tendon of FDP on its way to the base of the distal phalynx. The long flexors act upon the interphalangeal joints. Arising in the palm from the tendons of FDP are four palmar muscles known as the lumbricals which provide flexion at the metacarpal-phalyngeal joints. The lumbrical muscles are situated superficially to the interosseous muscles which fill the spaces between the metacarpals.

4

ABDOMEN

Q1

a Name the structure labelled A
b Name the structure labelled B
c Name the structure labelled C
d Name the structure labelled D
e Name the structure labelled E

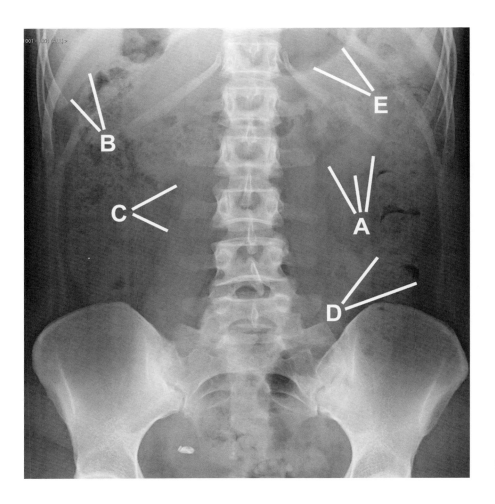

Q2

a Name the structures labelled A
b Name the structures labelled B
c Name the structure that partially arises from the antero-medial aspect of the structures labelled B
d Name the structure labelled D
e Name the skeletal anatomical variant demonstrated in this image

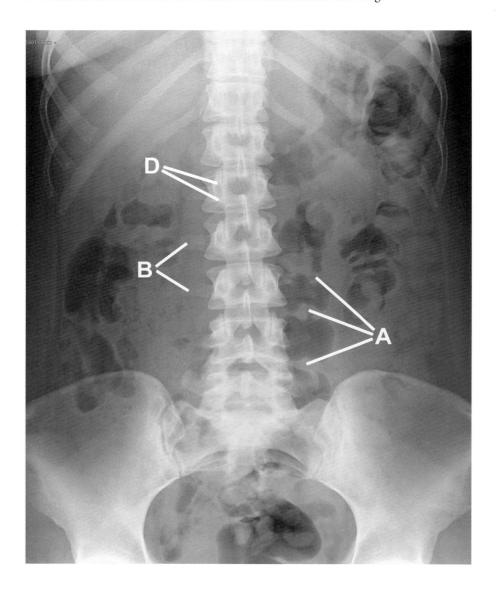

Q3

a Name the superficial blood vessel into which catheter A has been inserted
b Name the superficial blood vessel into which catheter B has been inserted
c Name the vessels/structures through which the tip of catheter A has travelled
d Name the vessels/structures through which the tip of catheter B has travelled
e Name the structure labelled E

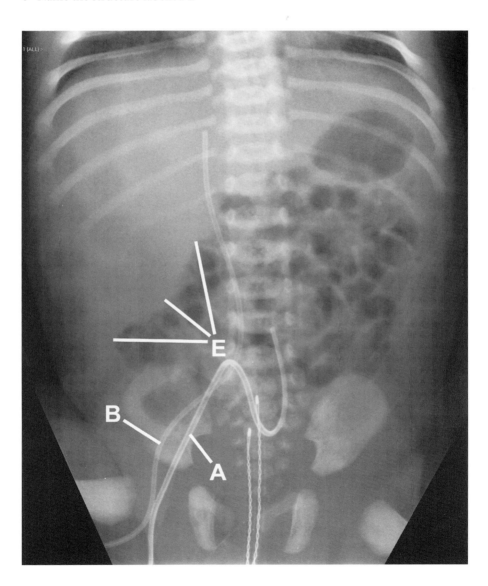

Q4

a Name the structure labelled A
b Name the vertebral column in which structure A lies
c Name the opening labelled C
d Name the structure labelled D
e Describe why structure D is atypical at the vertebral level indicated

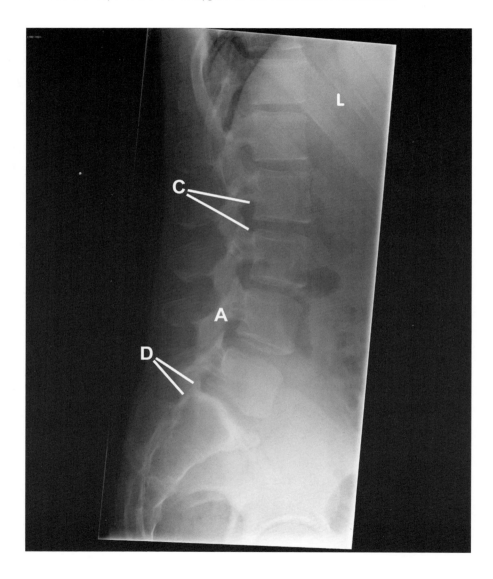

Q5

a Name the structure labelled A
b Name the structure labelled B
c Name the structure labelled C
d Name the structure labelled D
e Name the structure labelled E

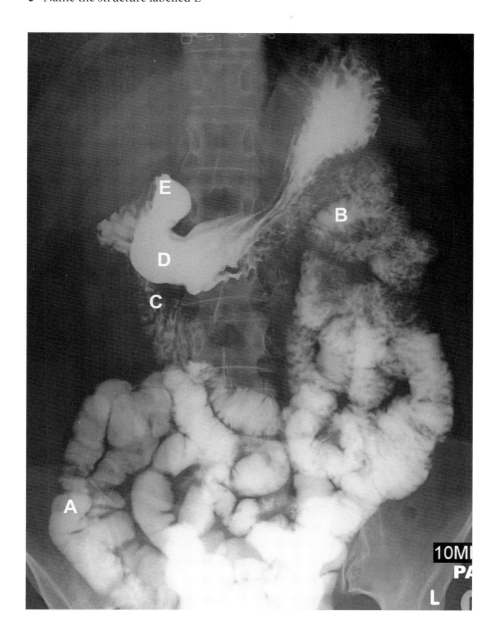

Q6

a Name the structure labelled A
b Name the structure labelled B
c Name the structure labelled C
d Name the structure labelled D
e Name the structure labelled E

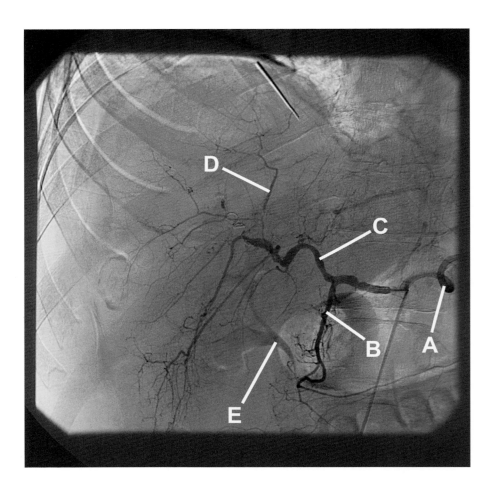

Q7

a Name the structure labelled A
b Name the structure labelled B
c Name the structure labelled C
d Name the structure labelled D
e Name the structure labelled E

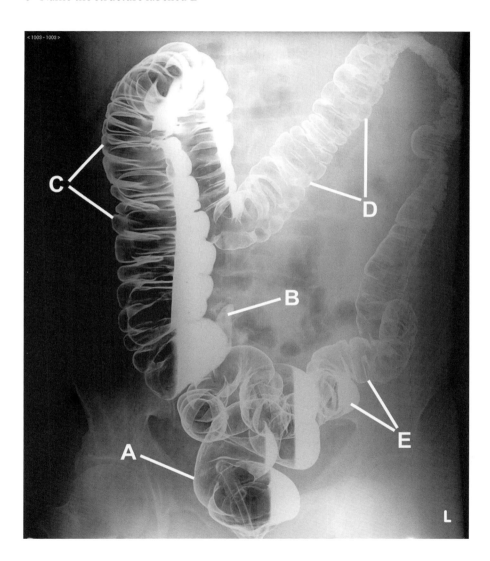

Q8

a Name the structure labelled A
b Name the structure labelled B
c Name the structure labelled C
d Name the structure labelled D
e Name the structure labelled E

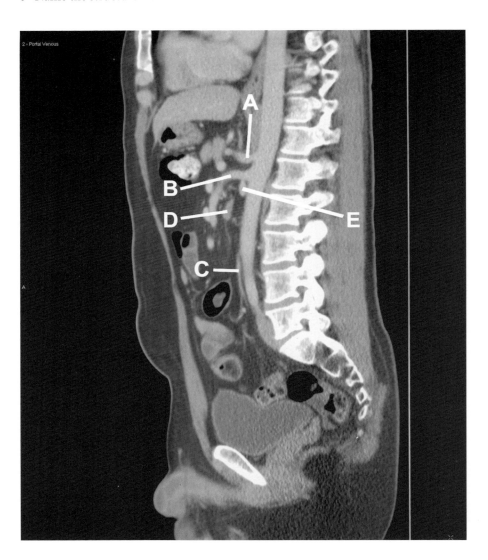

Q9

a Name the segment of the structure labelled A
b Name the segment of the structure labelled B
c Name the structure labelled C
d Name the structure labelled D
e Name the structure labelled E

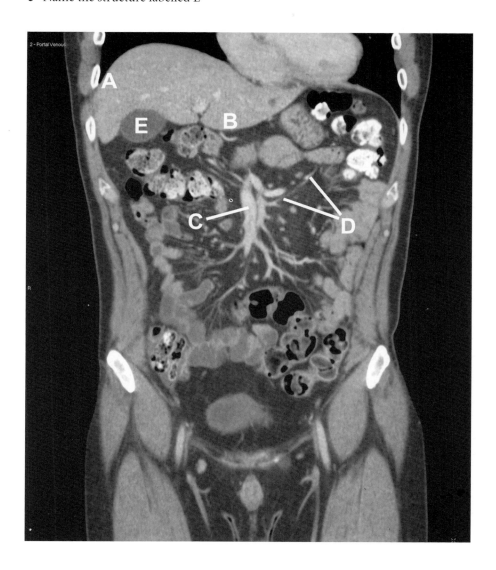

Q10

a Name the structure labelled A
b Name the structure labelled B
c Name the structure labelled C
d Name the structure labelled D
e Name the structure labelled E

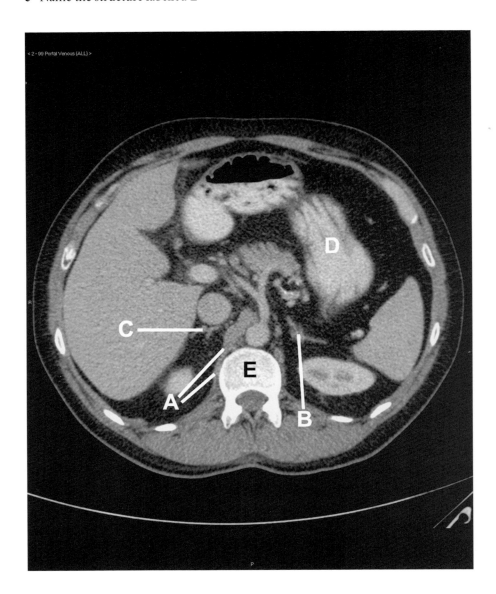

< 2 - 99 Portal Venous (ALL) >

Q11

a Name the peritoneal ligament arising from structure A
b Name the structure labelled B
c Name the structure labelled C
d Name the structure labelled D
e Name the peritoneal ligament arising from structure E

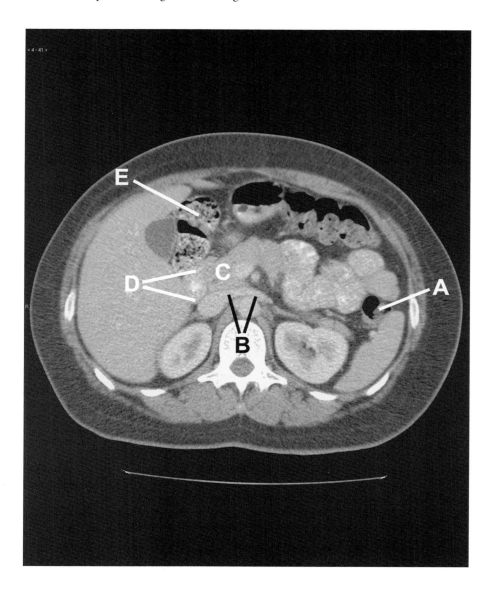

Q12

a Name the opening outlined and labelled A
b Name the cavity into which A opens
c Name the structure labelled C
d Name the peritoneal structure indicated by the lines labelled D
e Name the peritoneal structure indicated by the line labelled E

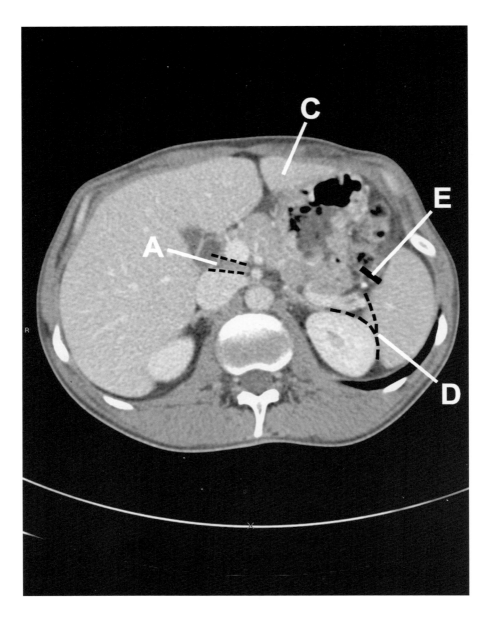

Q13

a Name the gas filled structure labelled A
b Name the structure labelled B
c Name the structure labelled C
d Name the structure labelled D
e Name the embryological vascular remnant located at site E

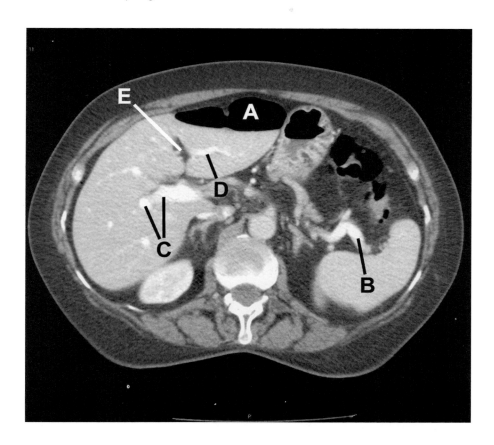

Q14

a Name the structure labelled A
b Name the structure labelled B
c Name the space labelled C
d Name the structure labelled D
e Name the anatomical variant demonstrated in this image

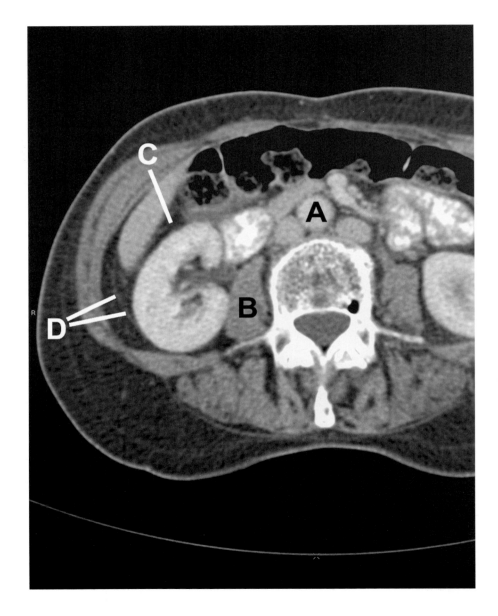

Q15

a Name the structure labelled A
b Name the region outlined and labelled B
c Name the structure labelled C
d Name the structure labelled D
e Name the structure responsible for the indentation at position E

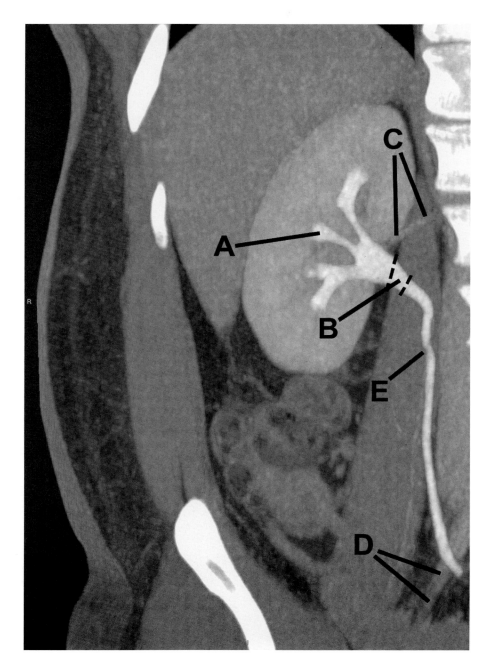

Q16

a Name the structure labelled A
b Name the structure labelled B
c Name the structure labelled C
d Name the structure labelled D
e Name the structure labelled E

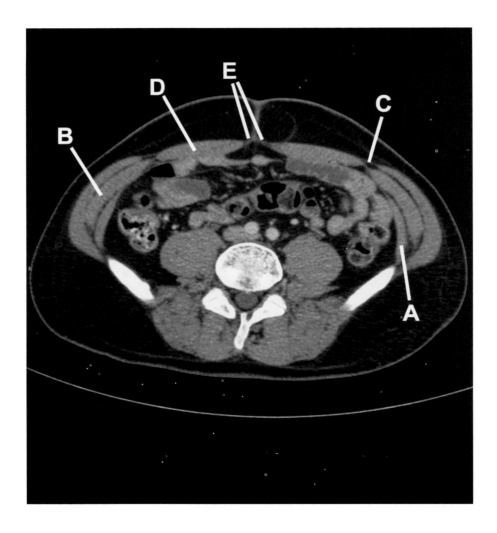

Q17

a Name the structure labelled A
b Name the structure labelled B
c Name the structure labelled C
d Name the structure labelled D
e Name the structure labelled E

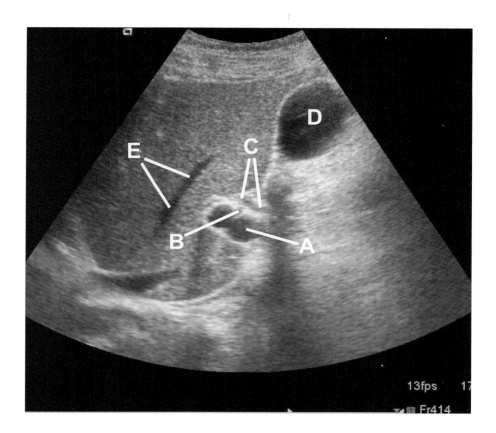

Q18

a   Name the structure labelled A
b   Name the structure labelled B
c   Name the part of the structure labelled C
d   Name the structure labelled D
e   Name the part of the structure labelled E

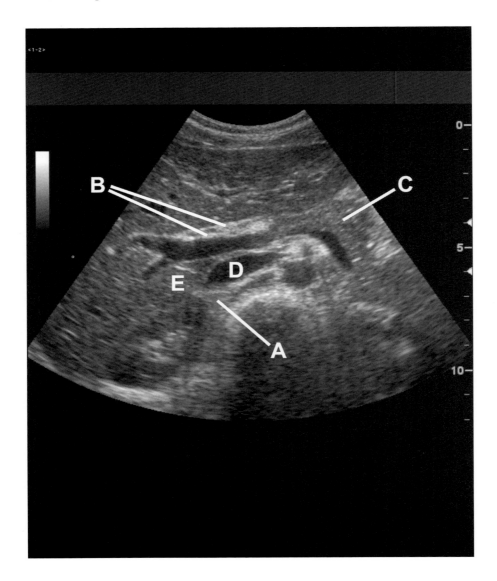

Q19

a Name the structure labelled A
b Name the structure labelled B
c Name the structure labelled C
d Name the structure labelled D
e Name the structure labelled E

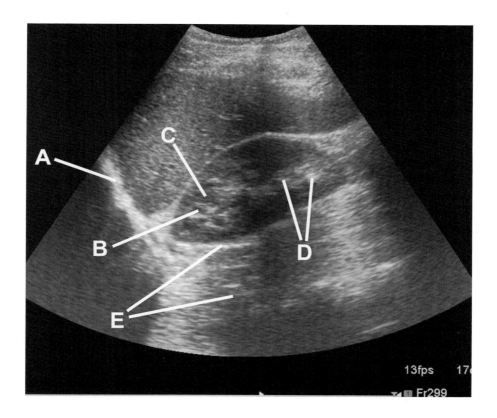

Q20

a Name the structure labelled A
b Name the structure labelled B
c Name the structure labelled C
d Name the major biliary structure not seen in this image
e Name the pancreatic anatomical variant demonstrated in this image

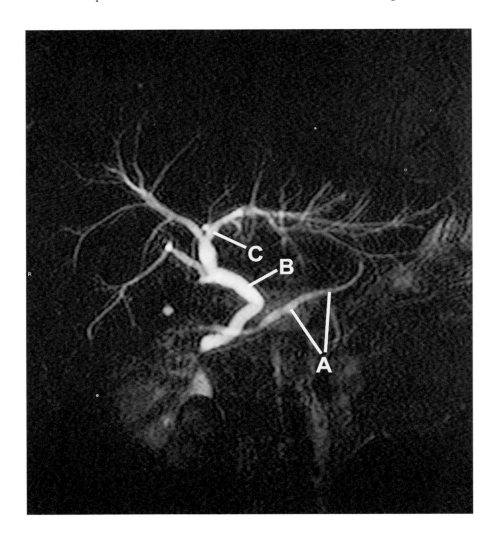

Q21

a Name the structure labelled A
b Name the structure labelled B
c Name the structure labelled C
d Name the structure labelled D
e Name the artery that supplies most of the spinal cord visible in this image (inferior to T9)

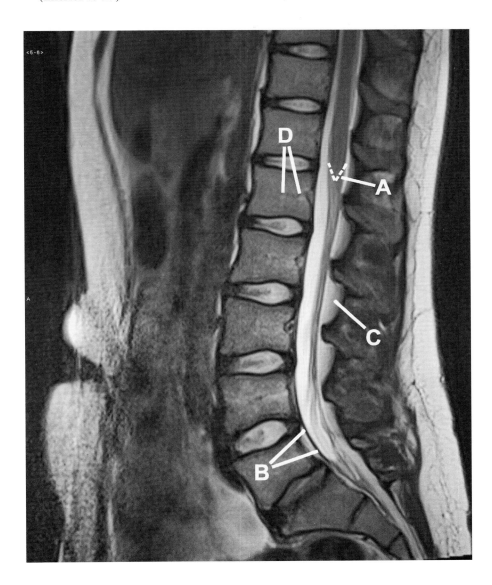

ABDOMEN – ANSWERS

Q1 Answers

a Left kidney
b Liver
c Right psoas muscle
d Descending colon
e Stomach

Abdominal radiograph

On plain radiography, the presence of an interface between tissues of differing contrast is required to enable visualization of structures. In the case of the liver, kidney and psoas muscles there is para-renal, peri-renal and retroperitoneal fat to provide this contrast. The descending colon is surrounded on three sides by peritoneum but there is adjacent preperitoneal fat which can give contrast, as in this case. There is often gas within the lumen of the bowel to provide negative contrast as is commonly seen in the stomach and colon.

Q2 Answers

a Haustra
b Transverse processes of lumbar spine
c Psoas major muscle
d Right pedicle of L2
e Six lumbar vertebrae (or one pre-sacral vertebra)

Abdominal radiograph

The teniae coli run the length of the colon, from the caecum to the sigmoid. They are focal areas of thickening in the longitudinal muscular layer which run along the anterior, postero-medial and postero-lateral aspects of the colon. As they are shorter than the colon, the bowel is pulled into folds, or haustra, which can be seen on radiographs. The taeniae coli converge at the appendix base proximally and the rectum distally.

The psoas major muscle arises from the antero-medial aspect of the lumbar transverse processes and the lower borders of the T12–L5 vertebral bodies.

Aberrations at the lumbar-sacral junction are occasionally seen. An example is the presence of six lumbar vertebrae, the sixth vertebra being called the first pre-sacral vertebra. 'Sacralization' of L5 occurs when it is fused to S1. 'Lumbarization' of S1, which is less common, occurs when S1 is significantly separated from S2.

Q3 Answers

a Left umbilical artery
b Umbilical vein
c Umbilical, left internal iliac and left common iliac arteries, aorta
d Umbilical vein, left portal vein, ductus venosus, IVC
e Liver

Abdominal radiograph of a neonate

Umbilical vascular catheters can be used for vascular sampling and monitoring in the neonatal period.

There are paired umbilical arteries which are branches of the internal iliac arteries on both sides. The distal artery will normally occlude shortly after transection of the cord at birth, going on to form the medial umbilical ligament. The proximal artery will remain patent however and provides branches to the bladder and ductus deferens. Early in-utero there is a pair of umbilical veins but only one usually persists to birth. This umbilical vein carries oxygenated blood towards the foetal heart and initially drains into the left portal vein, where it then bypasses the hepatic circulation to enter the inferior vena cava (IVC) through the ductus venosum. Both the ductus venosum and umbilical vein occlude and become fibrotic following birth, becoming the ligamentum venosum and ligamentum teres respectively.

The relative size of the normal liver is large in neonates. Proportional to total body height, the longitudinal length of the right lobe in neonates is almost twice that at aged 16 years.

Konuş OL, Ozdemir A, Akkaya A *et al.* Normal liver, spleen, and kidney dimensions in neonates, infants, and children: evaluation with sonography. *Am J Roentgenol* 1998; 171:1693–1698.

Q4 Answers

a Pars interarticularis
b Posterior column
c Neural foramen/intervertebral foramen
d Facet (zygapophyseal) joint
e The inferior articular facet faces forward

Radiograph of lumbar spine, lateral view

The anatomy of the five lumbar vertebrae differs from the thoracic vertebrae in a number of areas, enabling them to withstand greater degrees of axial stress. The vertebral bodies are larger in transverse diameter than in antero-posterior diameter. The adjacent articular facets directly face each other (in the sagittal plane) and the laminae are shorter and do not overlap. The pars interarticularis is the laminar region between the facet joints and is the area fractured in spodylolysis. The pedicles enclose the intervertebral or neural foramina, as happens in the thoracic spine.

The fifth lumbar vertebra is atypical of others, and has differences in structure to facilitate articulation with the sacrum. The vertebral body is wedge-shaped and is taller anteriorly to accommodate the downward sloping S1. The inferior facet faces forward which allows a stronger articulation with S1 and also prevents anterior subluxation. The transverse process is very large and triangular and attaches to the pedicle and vertebral body of L5.

The 'three column' principle can be used as a means of predicting mechanical integrity (and therefore the degree of stability) of the spine following injury or disruption.

- The anterior column is formed by the anterior longitudinal ligament, anterior part of the vertebral body and the anterior annulus fibrosis.
- The middle column consists of the posterior longitudinal ligament, posterior wall of the vertebral body and posterior annulus fibrosis.
- The posterior column consists of the neural arch (or posterior elements) and the posterior ligamentous complex of ligamentum flavum, interspinous ligaments, supraspinous ligaments and intertransverse ligaments.

Denis F. The three column spine and its significance in the classification of acute thoracolumbar spinal fractures. *Spine* 1983; 8:817–831.

Q5 Answers

a Ileum
b Jejunum
c Descending/second part of duodenum
d Gastric (pyloric) antrum
e Duodenal cap

Barium small bowel follow-through examination

The antrum of the stomach is the area distal to the incisura on the lesser curve and narrows to form the pyloric canal. The duodenum, which is mainly retroperitoneal, is roughly 'C'-shaped with the concavity to the left and is described in four parts. The first part of the duodenum travels posteriorly and superiorly to vertebral level L1, making it appear shortened in a frontal projection. Mucosal folds are thin and lie in a parallel or spiral configuration. The duodenal cap is the proximal 2.5cm of duodenum, which lies between the peritoneal folds of the greater and lesser omenta and forms the inferior boundary of the opening into the lesser sac (epiploic foramen). The second part of the duodenum runs inferiorly to vertebral level L3, and is where circular valvulae conniventes of small bowel begin properly. A longitudinal duodenal fold may be seen which marks the position of the ampulla (of Vater). The third part travels horizontally and the fourth part ascends to vertebral level L2 where it passes out from behind the peritoneum to become the jejunum at the duodenal-jejunal flexure. The ligament of Treitz is a thin musculofibrous suspensory band that connects the fourth part of the duodenum with the right diaphragmatic crus.

The proximal two-fifths of the small bowel is called the jejunum, the distal three-fifths the ileum. When compared to the ileum, the jejunum is usually of wider caliber, with a thicker wall and thicker, more numerous valvulae conniventes. The jejunum is usually positioned in the upper left abdomen, while the ileum lies in the lower right abdomen. In barium studies, the jejunum often shows a 'feathery' mucosal pattern, compared to a more solid and featureless appearance of the ileum.

Q6 Answers

a Splenic artery
b Gastroduodenal artery
c Common hepatic artery
d Left hepatic artery
e Right renal pelvis

Digital subtraction angiogram of the coeliac axis, AP view

The coeliac artery is the uppermost of three un-paired aortic branches which provide blood supply to the abdominal viscera. It arises from the anterior aspect of the abdominal aorta at the level of T12–L1 as a single trunk which typically branches into three divisions: the common hepatic, left gastric and splenic arteries which course right, superiorly and left respectively (the left gastric artery is not well opacified on this image). This usual configuration of vessels is present in around 55% of the population.

The coeliac trunk is primarily responsible for supplying the foregut structures, the superior mesenteric artery supplying the mid-gut and the inferior mesenteric artery the hindgut. In reality there are often rich vascular connections between these circulations and overlap of the territories they supply. There is a lot of variety in coeliac arterial anatomy amongst individuals. Michel's classification of hepatic arterial supply alone lists ten different normal variations.

Intra-arterial contrast is readily filtered from the blood by the kidneys once it enters the systemic circulation. Opacification of the renal collecting systems is commonly seen during angiographic studies.

Michel NA. *Blood supply and anatomy of the upper abdominal organs with a descriptive atlas*, Lippincott, Philadelphia, 1955, pp. 64–69.

Q7 Answers

a Rectum
b Appendix
c Ascending colon
d Transverse colon
e Sigmoid colon

Full length radiograph from a barium enema examination, frontal view

The large intestine consists of eight parts which, from proximal to distal, are: caecum, vermiform appendix, ascending colon, transverse colon, descending colon, sigmoid colon, rectum and anal canal.

The caecum is the blind-ended pouch of the colon just distal to the ileocaecal valve. It is covered with peritoneum which is reflected downwards to the floor of the right iliac fossa and determines both the mobility of the caecum and size of the retrocaecal space. The ascending and descending colon are invested in peritoneum and are relatively immobile. The transverse and sigmoid colon are invested in their own mesentery (or mesocolon), as is the appendix which arises from the posterior aspect of the caecum. These three are therefore the most mobile parts of the large intestine. The rectum is covered on its upper third by peritoneum. Deep to the peritoneal reflection, the rectum is surrounded by pelvic visceral fat and fascia (mesorectum).

Q8 Answers

a Coeliac trunk
b Superior mesenteric artery (SMA)
c Inferior mesenteric artery
d Third part of duodenum
e Left renal vein

Contrast enhanced abdomino-pelvic CT, midline sagittal section

This image demonstrates the relative positions of the three un-paired ventral aortic branches.

The coeliac trunk arises at the T12–L1 level and often takes a caudal course from the anterior aorta. It runs above the pancreas and the splenic vein and lies posterior to the left lobe of liver.

The SMA arises from the anterior aorta at around the level of L1. In approximately 0.5% of people the coeliac artery and SMA arise from a single (coeliacomesenteric) trunk. Running in a transverse direction deep to the SMA are the left renal vein and third part of duodenum. The pancreas and portal vein lie anteriorly. The SMA runs within the mesenteric root lying to the left of the superior mesenteric vein (SMV).

The inferior mesenteric artery (IMA) arises from the left anterior aspect of the

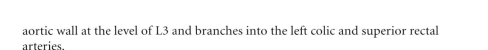

aortic wall at the level of L3 and branches into the left colic and superior rectal arteries.

Q9 Answers

a Right lateral superior (VII)
b Left medial inferior (III)
c Superior mesenteric vein
d Jejunal branch of the superior mesenteric artery
e Gallbladder

CT of abdomen and pelvis at the level of the superior mesenteric vessels, coronal section

The superior mesenteric artery arises just proximal to the origins of the renal arteries. The artery courses anteriorly and then inferiorly, running alongside and to the left of the superior mesenteric vein. From the left lateral aspect of the SMA, a total of 4–6 jejunal branches arise, with each artery dividing into two and joining to form an arcade of vessels which parallels the orientation of the intestine. A branch of the dorsal pancreatic artery may arise from the SMA just proximal to the first jejunal branch. The middle colic branch and right colic branch arise from the right side of the SMA, and supply the transverse colon and ascending colon respectively. Occasionally a second artery accompanies the middle colic artery in the transverse mesocolon before coursing inferiorly to connect with the left colic artery. This is known as an artery of Riolan and, if present, forms a communication between the superior mesenteric and inferior mesenteric arterial systems. The ileocolic artery arises from the distal SMA and supplies branches to the caecum, terminal ileum and appendix. A total of 9–13 ileal branches arise from the terminal SMA and form into arcades (in a similar fashion to the jejunal branches) to supply the ileum. The distal ileal branch forms an anastomosis with the ileocolic artery.

Hepatic segments are regions of the liver that share a common blood supply (both hepatic arterial and portal venous) and biliary drainage. There are eight segments in total and they were first described by Couinaud, a French hepatobiliary surgeon, in 1957. The liver is divided by the principal plane into two anatomical halves and these are further sub-divided into four segments. The planes of segmental division are marked by the hepatic veins in the longitudinal axis and the portal vein in the transverse axis. Segment IV is different in that it extends either side of the portal vein and can be given the suffix (a) for the superior part and (b) for the inferior part. When the liver is viewed from the front the segments are numbered in an approximately clockwise fashion beginning at the caudate lobe which is segment I. Segments VII, VIII, IV(a) and II run right-to-left superior to the portal vein and segments VI, V, IV(b) and III run in a similar manner inferior to the portal vein.

Claude Couinaud. *Le Foie: Études anatomiques et chirurgicales (The Liver: Anatomical and Surgical Studies)*, Masson, Paris, 1957.

Q10 Answers

a Crus of right hemi-diaphragm
b Left adrenal gland
c Right adrenal gland
d Body of the stomach
e T12 vertebral body

CT of the upper abdomen with oral and intravenous contrast, in the portal venous phase, axial section

The adrenal glands lie retroperitoneally and above the kidneys with the position of the gland on the right being more consistent. It lies posterior to the inferior vena cava, medial to the right lobe of the liver and lateral to the right diaphragmatic crus. It is lower and more medial in relation to the spine than the left adrenal.

The stomach is J-shaped and shows much variation in size and shape between individuals. It has two curvatures – the greater and lesser curves. The incisura is an angulation towards the pyloric end of the lesser curve. There are two orifices, the cardia (upper) and pylorus (lower). The part above the cardia is called the fundus. Between the cardia and the incisura is the body of the stomach and distal to the incisura is the gastric (pyloric) antrum. The stomach is lined by mucosa which forms into temporary folds called rugae. These can be seen in this image as lines running the length of the gastric body.

Q11 Answers

a Phrenicocolic ligament
b Left renal vein
c Head of pancreas
d Second part of duodenum
e Duodenocolic ligament

Porto-venous CT at the level of the L2 vertebra, axial section

The ascending and descending colon are both retroperitoneal structures which are fixed anteriorly and on both sides by peritoneum. At the hepatic flexure, the peritoneum extends to form the duodenocolic ligament which is continuous with the transverse mesocolon and contains the lymphatic vessels draining the right colon. The phrenicocolic ligament is a similar structure on the left side which extends from the splenic flexure to the diaphragm at the level of the 11th rib. This is continuous with both the transverse mesocolon and splenorenal ligament and provides additional support to the spleen as well as forming a barrier between the infracolic and supracolic compartments.

The left renal vein is five times longer than the right and passes anterior to the aorta from the renal hilum to drain into the IVC. It receives the inferior phrenic, gonadal and suprarenal veins on the left. The right renal vein receives no extrarenal tributaries.

Q12 Answers

a Foramen of Winslow/epiploic foramen
b Lesser sac
c Left lobe of the liver
d Splenorenal ligament
e Gastrosplenic ligament

CT abdomen at the level of L1, axial section

The lesser sac of the peritoneum lies between the pancreas and the posterior wall of the stomach, duodenum, lesser omentum and hepatoduodenal ligament. It extends for a variable extent superiorly to the diaphragmatic crus and inferiorly to the root of the transverse mesocolon. A fold of peritoneum surrounding the left gastric artery forms a division between two recesses in the lesser sac. The sac is formed from the embryological liver migrating from a central position into the right upper abdomen. This causes stretching of the visceral peritoneal covering and the creation of a space along its path.

The foramen of Winslow, or epiploic foramen, is a communication under the free bottom edge of the lesser omentum between the greater sac and lesser sac. It measures 25mm and is located between the IVC and free margin of the ligament containing the portal triad of vessels – the hepatoduodenal ligament.

The splenorenal, or lienorenal, ligament connects the posterior aspect of the spleen to the anterior para-renal space and contains the splenic vessels, tail of the pancreas and surrounding fat. The gastrosplenic ligament connects the greater curve of the stomach with the splenic hilum and contains left gastroepiploic and short gastric vessels. Together these two ligaments comprise the lateral boundary of the lesser sac.

DeMeo JH, Fulcher AS, Austin RF Jr *et al*. Anatomic CT demonstration of the peritoneal spaces, ligaments, and mesenteries: normal and pathologic processes. *Radiographics* 1995; 15:755–770.

Q13 Answers

a Transverse colon
b Splenic vein
c Right portal vein
d Left portal vein
e Umbilical vein

Upper abdominal CT with contrast (portal venous phase), axial section

The portal venous system serves to channel the blood drained from the gut and spleen into the liver prior to it entering the systemic circulation. The main portal vein is approximately 7cm long and is a direct continuation of the SMV, coursing anterior to the IVC towards the porta hepatis. Portal venous tributaries are the splenic (into which drains the inferior mesenteric vein), cystic, gastric and superior pancreatoduodenal veins. The portal vein divides into right and left limbs which in turn supply branches to the various hepatic segments. The portal vein supplies approximately 75% of the blood to the liver with the remainder being supplied via the hepatic arterial system.

Flow in the umbilical vein usually ceases following birth, but it remains a potential site of porto-systemic anastomoses. Other sites of porto-systemic anastomoses are at the lower oesophagus, upper anal canal, bare area of liver and retroperitoneal areas.

Q14 Answers

a Abdominal aorta
b Psoas muscle
c Hepato-renal (Morison's) pouch
d Posterior renal fascia (fascia of Zuckerlandl)
e Double IVC

Abdominal CT with oral and IV contrast, axial section

The IVC is normally formed from the confluence of the common iliac veins at the L5 level, behind the right common iliac artery and it travels up the posterior abdominal wall on the right of the midline. Developmental anomalies of one or more of the caval segments (hepatic, supra-renal, renal and infra-renal) are occasionally present. Duplication of the infra-renal IVC ('Double-IVC') is a developmental anomaly of the infra-renal segment resulting in persistence of both embryological supracardinal veins and is seen in 0.2–3% of the population. In these cases the left IVC typically drains into the left renal vein, which in turn joins the right-sided IVC as normal. Variations in the configuration of the renal segment (right suprasubcardinal and postsubcardinal anastomoses) are most common anomalies encountered, with retro-aortic and circum-aortic left renal veins present in approximately 8% and 2% of the population, respectively.

The kidneys are surrounded by perirenal fat which in turn is surrounded by the anterior and posterior leaves of renal fascia. The anterior leaf is Gerota's fascia and the posterior leaf is the fascia of Zuckerlandl. These divide the retroperitoneal space into three compartments: the peri-renal, anterior para-renal and posterior-para-renal spaces.

Morison's pouch lies at the posterior aspect of the right sub-hepatic space anterior to the right kidney and is the most dependant position of the peritoneal cavity in a supine patient. Its importance as a potential site of fluid accumulation within the abdomen was described by Morison in 1894.

Bass JE, Redwine MD, Kramer LA *et al.* Spectrum of Congenital Anomalies of the Inferior Vena Cava: Cross-sectional Imaging Findings. *RadioGraphics* 2000; 20:639–652.

Cheesbrough RM. Gerota versus Zuckerkandl: the renal fascia revisited. *Radiology* 1989; 173:845–846.

Morison JR. The Anatomy of the Right Hypochondrium Relating Especially to Operations for Gall Stones. 1894; 1766:968–971.

Q15 Answers

a Major calyx
b Pelvi-ureteric junction
c Renal artery
d External iliac artery
e Gonadal artery

CT urogram of the right kidney, maximum intensity projection, coronal section

The renal collecting system consists of several minor calyces which form two or three major calyces. These then drain into the renal pelvis, which is a conical structure located at the hilum of the kidney. It is usually the most posterior of the hilar structures. The right renal artery is longer than the left and the opposite is true with the renal veins. The kidney consists of five segments (apical, posterior, lower, upper and middle) which are each supplied by a segmental artery and vein.

The transition between renal pelvis and ureter is the pelvi-ureteric junction, which along with the vesico-ureteric junction are the narrowest segments of the upper renal tract.

The ureter passes inferiorly along the anterior border of psoas major muscle. It is crossed by the gonadal artery which arises from the anterior aorta (L2 vertebral level) and travels obliquely down towards the testis or ovaries. Inferiorly the right ureter is crossed by the ileo-colic and right colic vessels as well as the root of the mesentery. It deviates medially from the psoas muscle and crosses anterior to the bifurcation of the common iliac artery (where the iliac artery is positioned anterior to the iliac vein) prior to passing into the pelvis.

Q16 Answers

a Transversus abdominis
b Internal oblique
c Aponeurosis of external oblique
d Rectus abdominis
e Linea alba

CT at the level of the iliac crest, axial section

The musculature of the anterior and lateral abdominal wall consists of four main muscles; rectus abdominis, external oblique, internal oblique and transversus abdominis.

The two recti lie either side of the midline and extend from the 5th, 6th and 7th costal cartilages to the pubis. They are interconnected by the linea alba and invested within a thick fascial covering known as the rectus sheath which is formed by the aponeuroses of the external oblique, internal oblique and transversus abdominis muscles.

The external oblique is the largest and most superficial of the three antero-lateral muscles. It arises from ribs 4–12 and interdigitates with slips of muscle from serratus anterior and latissimus dorsi. As it passes anteriorly it becomes an aponeurosis which forms part of the anterior rectus sheath, anterior to rectus abdominis. The free lower edge of the external oblique is attached between the anterior superior iliac spine and the pubic tubercle and forms the inguinal ligament.

The internal oblique lies deep to and is smaller than the external oblique. It arises from the costal margin and thoracolumbar fascia and is inserted into the inguinal ligament below. As it passes anteriorly it becomes an aponeurosis which, above the umbilicus, splits around the rectus abdominis and contributes to both the anterior and posterior layers of the rectus sheath.

The transversus abdominis is the deepest of the three muscles, arising from the costal margin, thoracolumbar fascia, iliac crest and inguinal ligament. It also becomes an aponeurosis which, above the umbilicus contributes to the posterior layer of the rectus sheath.

Below the umbilicus, all three aponeuroses pass anterior to the rectus abdominis. This produces a whitening of the anterior wall where the rectus passes deep to all three layers and is known as the arcuate line.

Q17 Answers

a Portal vein
b Hepatic artery
c Common bile duct
d Gallbladder
e Hepatic vein

Ultrasound of the liver at the porta-hepatis, transverse section

The common bile duct lies anterior to the portal vein at the porta-hepatis. To the left of the common bile duct and running in an oblique course, is the hepatic artery. The diameter of the common bile duct is measured at the level of the hepatic artery and should not exceed 4mm in young adults. The calibre of the common bile duct usually increases with age.

The portal veins characteristically have hyperechoic walls which can enable differentiation on ultrasound from dilated biliary ducts or hepatic veins, which typically do not. The venous drainage of the liver occurs directly into the IVC through the middle, left and right hepatic veins. They form a confluence with the intra-hepatic IVC at the level of T9, just below the caval diaphragmatic hiatus.

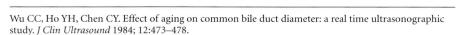

Wu CC, Ho YH, Chen CY. Effect of aging on common bile duct diameter: a real time ultrasonographic study. *J Clin Ultrasound* 1984; 12:473–478.

Laing FC. The gallbladder and bile ducts. In *Diagnostic ultrasound* (eds Rumack C, Wilson S, Carboneau JW), Mosby, St Louis, MO, 1998, p. 207.

Q18 Answers

a Right adrenal/supra-renal gland
b Common bile duct
c Body of the pancreas
d Inferior vena cava
e Caudate lobe (segment I) of the liver

Ultrasound of upper abdomen, transverse section

The right adrenal (supra-renal) gland lies antero-medial to the right upper pole of the kidney and it is adherent to the posterior wall of the inferior cava. The blood supply is principally provided by the suprarenal artery, however collateral supply comes from the renal and inferior phrenic arteries. Venous drainage is through the suprarenal vein, which drains into the IVC on the right and the left renal vein on the left. The adrenals are a similar size on both sides, with the average widths of the anterior, posteromedial and posterolateral limbs being 6.5mm, 3mm and 3mm respectively. The anterior limb of the right adrenal is usually less prominent than the left because of its proximity to the IVC.

The pancreas is divided into four parts – head, neck, body and tail. The head lies to the right of the midline and within the concavity of the duodenal curve and extends inferiorly as the hook-shaped uncinate process. The neck is the part of the pancreas which is immediately anterior to the proximal portal vein. The body begins in line with the left border of the vertebral column and the distal pancreatic tail is the part contained within the lienorenal ligament alongside the splenic vessels.

The caudate lobe (segment I) of the liver is situated posterior and to the right of the hepatic IVC. It is unusual in that it receives a blood supply from both right and left hepatic arteries and portal veins and drains directly into the IVC through small perforating veins.

Q19 Answers

a Right hemi-diaphragm
b Renal pyramid
c Column of Bertin
d Renal sinus fat
e Right psoas major

Ultrasound of right kidney, longitudinal section

The kidney parenchyma comprises of an outer cortex and inner medulla. Columns of Bertin are regions of cortical tissue which pass towards the renal hilum dividing the medulla into several pyramids. At the top of the pyramids, the papillae drain into the calyces which in turn drain into the renal pelvis. The renal sinus partially encloses the renal pelvis and contains fat and lymphatics.

The hemi-diaphragm is located above the kidney and has an echogenic appearance on ultrasound. Psoas major lies postero-medially and can be seen in longitudinal section below the kidney.

Q20 Answers

a Dorsal pancreatic duct (of Santorini)
b Common bile duct
c Left hepatic bile duct
d Gallbladder
e Pancreas divisum

MRCP

Bile drained from the hepatocytes runs in bile duct tributaries which pass alongside portal venous and hepatic arterial vessels in 'portal triads'. All three systems conform to the segmental divisions of the liver. The segmental and sectoral ducts typically unite to form the right and left hepatic ducts which then converge at the porta hepatis to become the common hepatic duct. The cystic duct from the gallbladder usually drains into the common hepatic duct, after which it becomes the common bile duct (CBD). The location of cystic duct insertion and therefore the length of the common bile duct can vary, however an average length is approximately 8cm.

There are numerous variations in the configuration and course of the intra-hepatic biliary ducts and in approximately 50% the anatomy is not 'typical' (as in this image). In this case the main confluence at the porta hepatis is formed by a right sectoral duct and the left hepatic duct, with the remaining right sectoral duct inserting more distally into the CBD. This is one of the convergence étagée or shelved confluence variations seen in approximately 20% of the population. This variation is of interest to surgeons as an aberrant posterior sectoral duct can be mistaken for the cystic duct during gallbladder surgery.

The gallbladder is not visible on this image. There can be a number of reasons for this which include: previous cholecystectomy (common), chronic cholecystitis, cholelithiasis and agenesis (rare).

Normally the pancreatic duct combines with the common bile duct to form the ampulla of Vater. This then drains into the second part of the duodenum, with the flow being controlled by a muscular sphincter (of Oddi). The main pancreatic duct is formed in-utero from fusion of the embryological dorsal and ventral ducts. It is common for some communication to persist between the pancreatic ductal systems but in approximately 6% of individuals these ducts remain entirely separate in what is termed pancreas divisum. In this anatomical variant the main dorsal duct (of Santorini) drains the tail and body of the pancreas and empties into the duodenum proximally via a separate opening – the minor papilla. The smaller ventral duct (of Wirsung), which serves the pancreatic head, then joins the distal CBD to drain into the duodenum via the major papilla. The ventral duct is seen on this image running inferior and parallel to the distal CBD.

Healy JE, Schroy PC. Anatomy of the Biliary Ducts Within the Human Liver: Analysis of the Prevailing Pattern of Branchings and the Major Variations of the Biliary Ducts. *AMA Arch Surg* 1953; 66:599–616.

Bismuth H, Vibert E. Chapter 90: Surgical Anatomy of the Liver and Biliary Ducts. In *Master Volume of Surgery, Volume 1* (eds Fischer JE, Bland KI), Lippincott Williams & Wilkins 2007.

Khan MA, Aktar A. Pancreas Divisum. *Radiology* 2010; eMedicine: www.emedicine.medscape.com

Q21 Answers

a Conus medullaris
b Posterior longitudinal ligament
c Epidural fat
d Basivertebral vein
e Artery of Adamkiewicz

T2W MRI of lower spine, midline sagittal section

The spinal cord terminates at the conus medullaris which is located opposite L1 or L2 in adults, but is positioned lower (L3) in children. This occurs because the relative growth of the spinal canal and meninges is greater than that of the spinal cord. The conus medullaris marks the termination of the cord only, as the lumbar and sacral nerve roots continue their descent within the thecal sac forming the cauda equina. There is a bulge in the spinal cord proximal to its termination, at around the level of T9–L1 vertebral bodies. This is the lumbar enlargement and is the location of the lower limb plexus (L2–S3) of nerve roots. A similar, but smaller, cervical enlargement occurs in the cord at the C3–T1 vertebral levels due to the upper limb plexus of nerve roots (C5–T1). Both of these enlargements occur as a result of a greatly increased mass of motor cells within the anterior horns of the grey matter.

The posterior longitudinal ligament provides stability to the posterior border of the vertebral bodies and intervertebral discs extending from the body of the axis (C2) to the sacrum. It is attached to the intervertebral discs but separated from the posterior wall of the vertebral bodies by the basivertebral veins and the associated venous plexus. The epidural space lies between the posterior longitudinal ligament and spinal dura. This space is more capacious in the lumbar region than elsewhere and is filled with epidural fat.

Blood supply to the spinal cord is through one anterior and two posterolateral spinal arteries. The proximal arteries supplying them vary throughout the length of the cord. Several radiculomedullary and intercostal arteries supply the upper (C1–T2) and middle (T3–T8) territories respectively, however the blood supply to the lower segment is mainly provided from a single source, the artery of Adamkiewicz. It usually arises from a radicular artery somewhere between the 9th thoracic and 1st lumbar segment and on the left side 80% of the time. The inconsistency in its location makes it susceptible to inadvertent iatrogenic damage during endovascular intervention. Two pairs of basivertebral veins drain each of the thoracic and lumbar vertebra and empty into the epidural plexus.

Q1

a Name the space labelled A
b Name the bony contour labelled B
c Name the muscle that attaches to C
d Name the bony structure labelled D
e Name the bony structure indicated as E

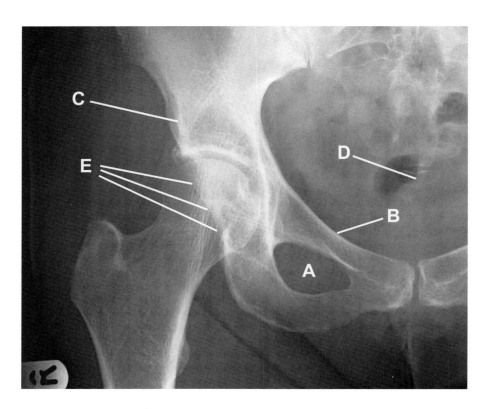

Q2

a Name the structure labelled A
b Name the structure labelled B
c Name the structure labelled C
d Name the structure labelled D
e Name the structures labelled E

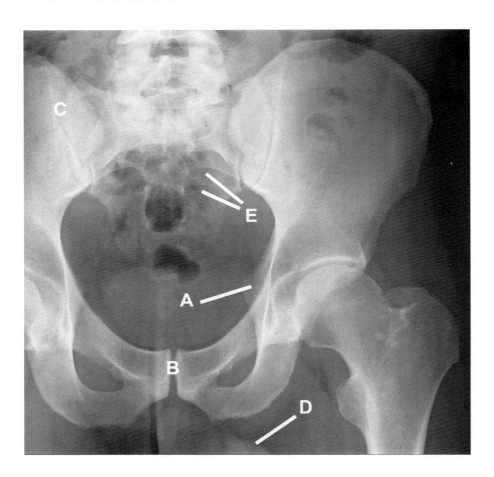

Q3

a Name the structure labelled A
b Name the structure labelled B
c Name the vessels over which the ureter crosses at the level labelled C
d Name the structure labelled D which is seen projected through the bladder
e Define the gender of this patient

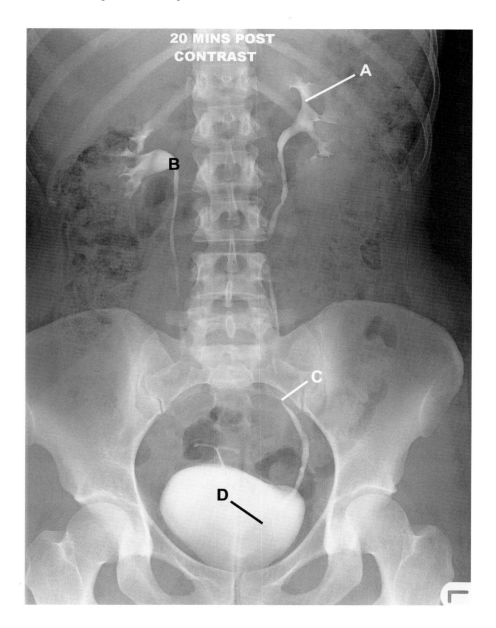

Q4

a Name the space indicated by A
b Name the structure labelled B
c Name the structure labelled C
d Name the structures labelled D
e Name the arteries supplying the rectum

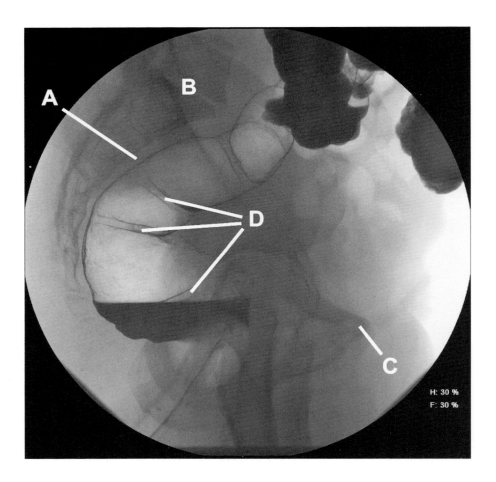

Q5

a Name the structure labelled A
b Name the structure labelled B
c Name the structure filled with gas and outlined by C
d Name the structure labelled D
e Name the structure labelled E

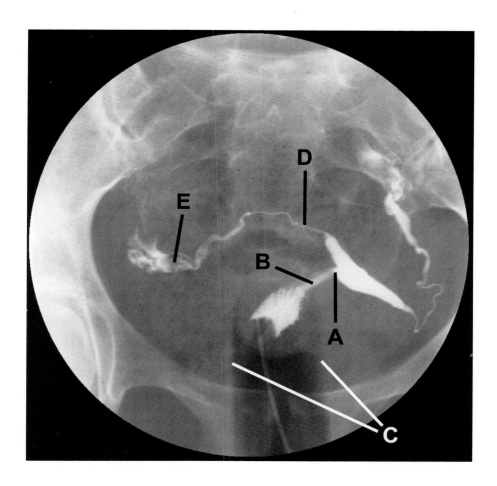

Q6

a Name the structure labelled A
b Name the structure labelled B
c Name the structure labelled C
d Name the structure labelled D
e Name the structure labelled E

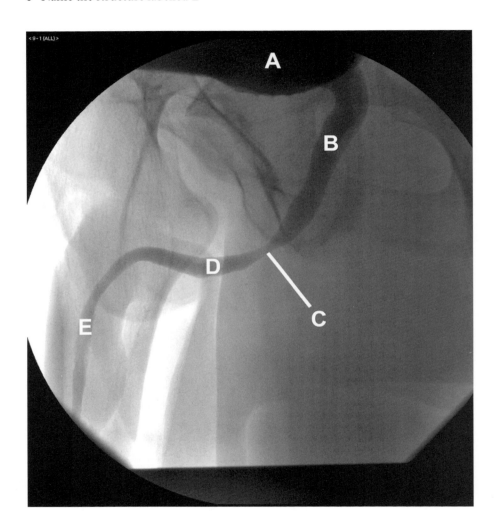

Q7

a Name the structure labelled A
b Name the structure labelled B
c Name the structure labelled C
d Name the structure labelled D
e Name the muscle group labelled E

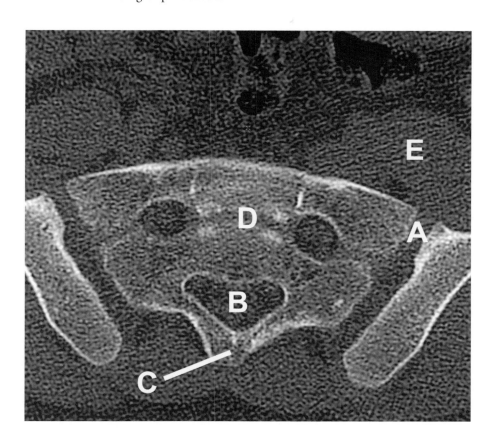

Q8

a Name the structure labelled A
b Name the structure labelled B
c Name the layer labelled C
d Name the layer labelled D
e Name the structure labelled E

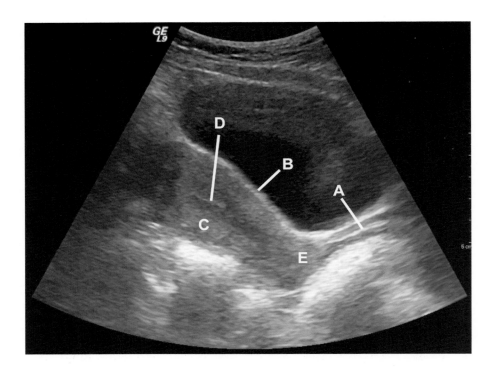

Q9

a Name the structure labelled A
b Name the structure labelled B
c Define CRL as labelled C
d Name the structure labelled D
e Name the structure labelled E

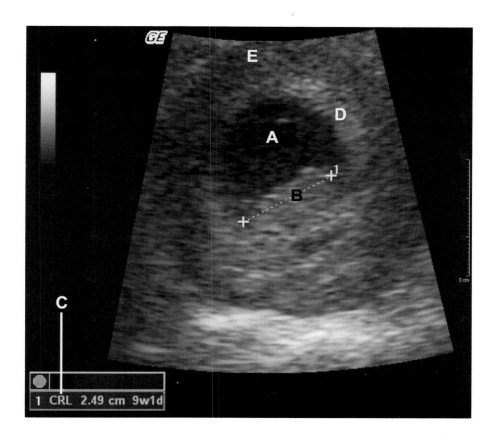

Q10

a Name the structure labelled A
b Name the structures labelled B
c Name the artery and vein normally found in the position labelled C
d Name the blood vessel from which arterial supply for A arises
e Name the three ligamentous attachments of A

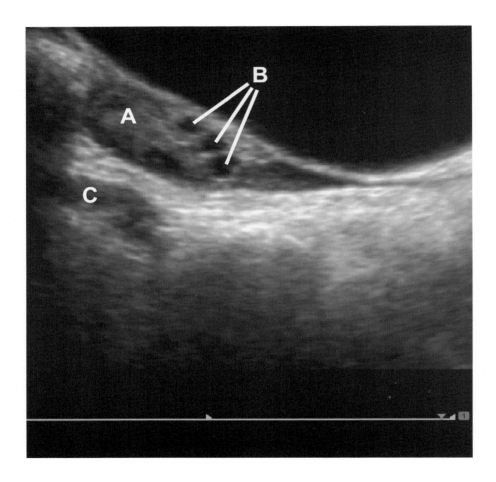

Q11

a Name the structure labelled A
b Name the structure labelled B
c Name the structure labelled C
d Name the structure labelled D
e Name the structure labelled E

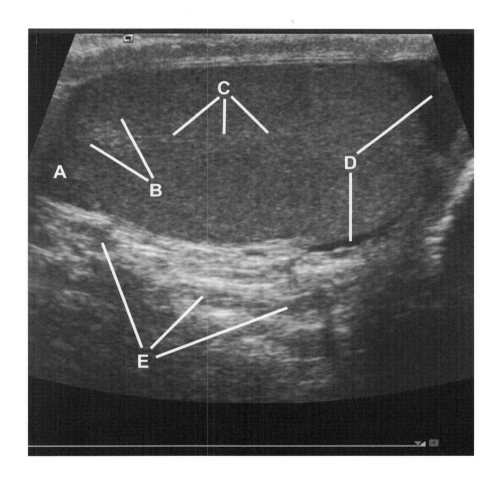

Q12

a Name the structure labelled A
b Name the structure labelled B
c Name the structure labelled C
d Name the structure labelled D
e Name the functional muscle group to which E belongs

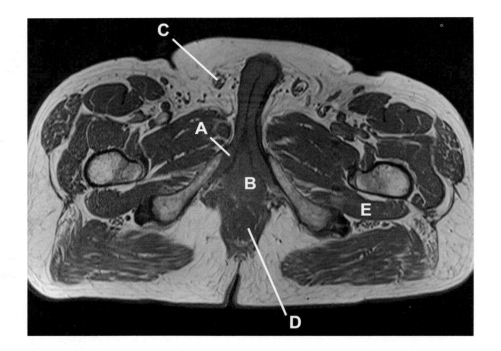

Q13

a   Name the structure labelled A
b   Name the structure labelled B
c   Name the structure labelled C
d   Name the structure labelled D
e   Name the structure labelled E

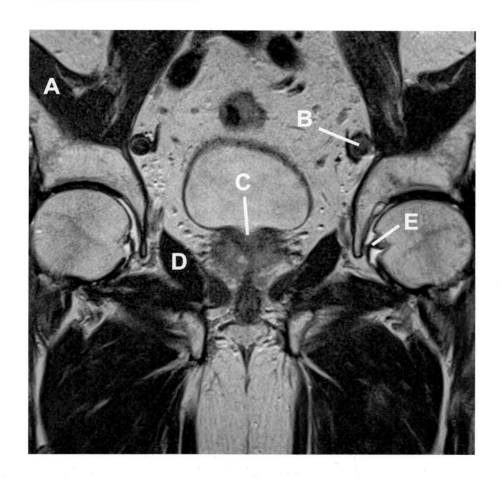

Q14

a Name the structure labelled A
b Name the structure labelled B
c Name the structure labelled C
d Name the structure labelled D
e Name the structure labelled E

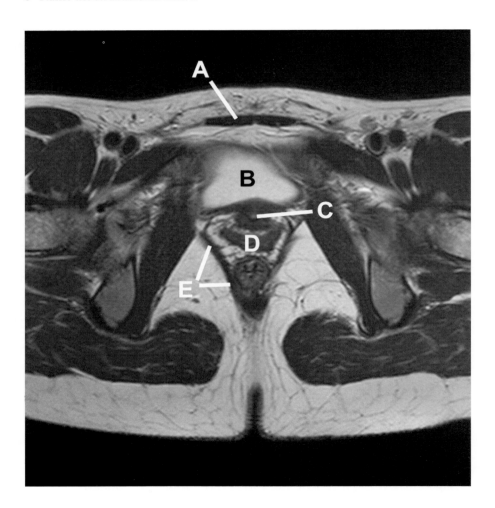

Q15

a Name the structure labelled A
b Name the structure labelled B
c Name the structure labelled C
d Name the structure labelled D
e Name the structure labelled E

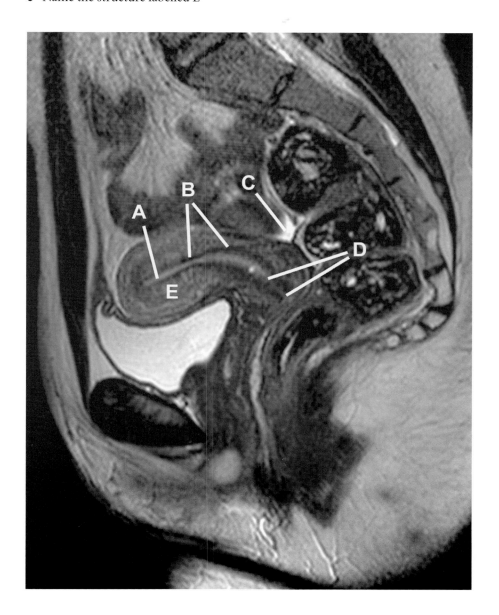

Q16

a Name the structure labelled A
b Name the structure labelled B
c Name the fatty spaces either side of structure B
d Name the structure labelled D
e Name the structure labelled E

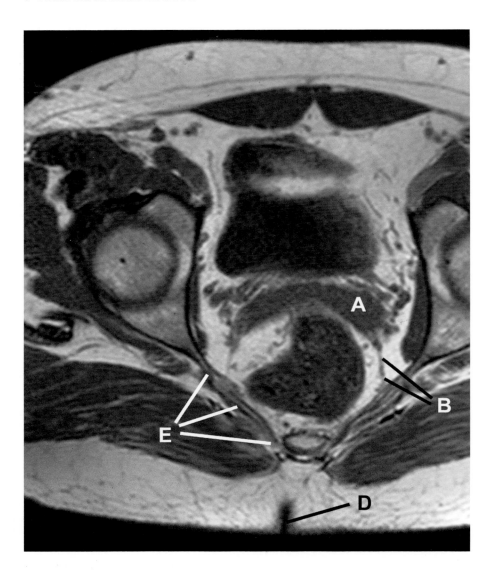

Q17

a Name the structure labelled A
b Name the structure labelled B
c Name the structure labelled C
d Name the structure labelled D
e Name the structure labelled E

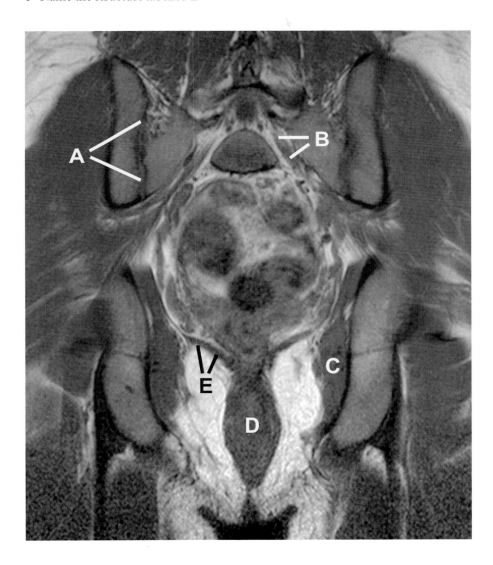

Q18

a Name the structure labelled A
b Name the structure labelled B
c Name the structure labelled C
d Name the structure labelled D
e Name the structure labelled E

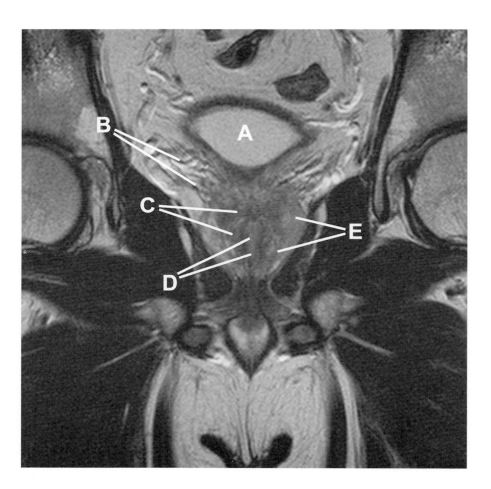

Q19

a Name the vertebral level at which the aorta bifurcates, as labelled A
b Name the artery labelled B
c Name the major divisions of the internal iliac artery
d Name one of the branches of the external iliac artery
e Name the vessel from which the gonadal arteries arise

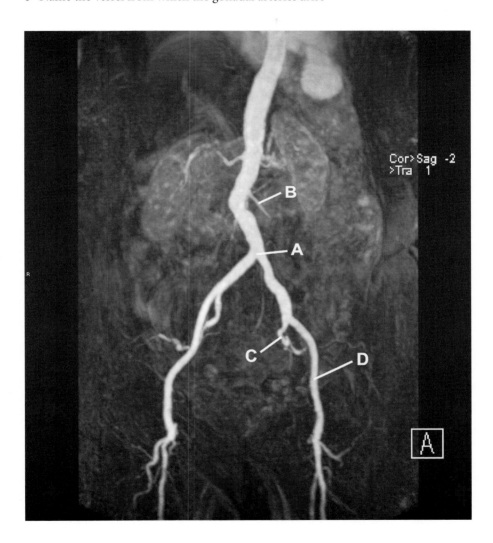

Q1 Answers

a Obturator foramen
b Pectineal line
c The straight head of rectus femoris attaches to the anterior inferior iliac spine
d Coccyx
e Posterior rim of right acetabulum

Radiograph of female pelvis, close up frontal view

The bony pelvis forms a complete ring and is composed of the paired innominate bones (themselves a fusion of three bones; ilium, ischium and pubis), the sacrum and coccyx. The paired sacro-iliac joints and pubic symphysis complete the ring.

The obturator foramina are almost completely closed over by the obturator membrane but do transmit the obturator nerves and vessels which supply the inner thigh.

Q2 Answers

a Ischial spine
b Pubic symphysis
c Sacro-iliac (SI) joint
d Soft tissue penile shadow
e Anterior sacral formina

Radiograph of male pelvis, close up frontal view

The morphology of the male and female pelvis differs in a number of ways. The male pelvis is more narrow and deep and it is said to be heart-shaped compared with the more round or oval, wide and shallow female pelvis. The sub-pubic angle formed by the pubic rami is more acute in the male pelvis and the ischial spines are usually more prominent. Soft tissue shadowing from genitalia or implantable contraceptive devices may give further clues as to the gender of the patient.

The sacral foramina allow passage of the sacral nerves and accompanying vessels.

Q3 Answers

a Upper pole major calyx
b Pelvi-ureteric junction (PUJ)
c Common iliac vessels
d Vesico-ureteric junction (VUJ)
e Female patient. Note an intra uterine contraceptive device is in situ. In addition, the bony pelvis has a classical female configuration

Intravenous Urogram (IVU), full length AP view

At the apex of the renal pyramids (renal papillae) formed urine drains into the cup-shaped minor renal calyces. These coalesce into two or sometimes three major calyces which further join to form the renal pelvis. The ureters are fibromuscular tubes which run from the renal pelvis (pelvi-ureteric junction, PUJ) to the postero-lateral aspect of the bladder (vesico-ureteric junction, VUJ). The ureters run along the posterior abdominal wall over the psoas muscle. At the pelvic brim they run anterior to the common iliac vessels; this causes a narrowing of the ureter seen on IVU which is projected at the level of the sacroiliac joints.

Q4 Answers

a Presacral space
b L5/S1 or lumbosacral joint
c Pubic tubercle
d Rectal folds or rectal valves
e Superior, middle and inferior rectal arteries

Lateral rectal view from barium enema series

The rectum is the terminal part of the colon. Anatomically the rectum follows the curves of the lower sacrum and coccyx when viewed laterally (as shown) and is S-shaped (when viewed in an AP projection). The three curves of this 'S' are represented internally as transverse folds known as the rectal valves (of Houston).

The presacral space contains fat, blood vessels, lymph nodes and lymphatics and also nerves.

The superior rectal artery represents the continuation of the inferior mesenteric artery and supplies the proximal rectum. The paired middle rectal arteries are branches of the anterior division of the internal iliac artery. The paired inferior rectal arteries are branches of the internal pudendal artery, which is also a branch of the anterior division of the internal iliac.

Q5 Answers

a Internal cervical ostium (internal os)
b Cervical canal
c Gas-filled vagina
d Isthmus of the fallopian tube
e Infundibulum of the fallopian tube

Normal hysterosalpingogram

When investigating female subfertility, uterine tubal patency can be assessed with a fluoroscopic hysterosalpingogram where contrast is passed into the uterine cavity. A normal result demonstrates unobstructed tubal flow and free spillage of contrast into the peritoneal cavity bilaterally. Identifiable features include the cervical canal between the external and internal ostia, a normally triangular-shaped uterine cavity, and the isthmus (narrowest part), ampulla (longest and widest mid portion) and infundibulum (funnel-shaped distal end sited in relation to the ovary) of the uterine (fallopian) tubes.

Sieglar AM. Hysterosalpingography. *Fertil Steril* 1983; 40:139–158.

Q6 Answers

a Urinary bladder filled with radio opaque contrast
b Prostatic urethra
c Membranous urethra
d Bulbous urethra
e Penile urethra

Micturating cystourethrogram in an adult male, oblique view

The male urethra is much longer than the female urethra. In general terms, the male urethra is divided into anterior and posterior segments. The posterior urethra runs from the internal (involuntary) sphincter at the bladder neck to the urogenital diaphragm (true pelvic floor) and includes prostatic and membranous parts. The membranous urethra is the narrowest part and represents the external (voluntary) sphincter where the urethra crosses the urogenital diaphragm. Distal to this, the anterior urethra (also known as the spongy urethra due to its course through corpus spongiosum) is composed of bulbous (within bulb of penis) and penile segments.

The ejaculatory ducts empty into the prostatic urethra.

Q7 Answers

a Sacro-iliac (SI) joint
b Sacral canal
c Median sacral crest
d Unfused S1–S2 joint
e Iliopsoas (hip flexors)

Oblique view of paediatric sacrum from CT study presented in bone windows

The sacrum forms from fusion of the five sacral vertebrae; this process is not complete until adulthood. Fusion of the spinous processes of the sacral vertebrae creates the median sacral crest. The sacral canal is a continuation of the vertebral canal and transmits the sacral nerve roots (cauda equina) which subsequently exit the sacrum via the anterior or posterior sacral foramina.

Q8 Answers

a Vaginal stripe (collapsed vaginal cavity)
b Bladder wall
c Myometrium
d Endometrium
e Cervix

Trans-abdominal ultrasound of the female pelvis, midline sagittal view

With trans-abdominal ultrasound of the female reproductive tract, the inferiorly placed vagina lies at an acute angle to the uterus (the latter is anteflexed over the bladder) and its cavity is usually collapsed appearing as an echogenic stripe. The thick muscular (myometrial) layer of the uterus appears less bright and is homogenous. Internal to this, the central endometrial stripe is also echogenic on ultrasound. The thickness of the endometrium changes according to the stage of the menstrual cycle; post menopause, endometrial thickening can indicate disease. The cervix forms the cylindrical inferior part of the uterus and provides communication between the vaginal and uterine cavities.

Q9 Answers

a Gestational sac
b Foetus
c Crown Rump Length
d Chorion
e Myometrium

Zoomed image from trans-abdominal ultrasound displaying early pregnancy

Ultrasound performed in early pregnancy can enable assessment of gestational age; this can be calculated using several means, but measurement of foetal crown-rump length (CRL) or biparietal diameter is common. The echobright layer surrounding the gestational sac is the chorion.

Campbell S, Warsof SL, Little D, Cooper DJ. Routine ultrasound screening for the prediction of gestational age. *Obstetrics & Gynaecology* 1985; 65:613–620.

Q10 Answers

a Ovary
b Developing ovarian follicles
c Internal iliac artery and vein
d Aorta
e Ligament of ovary, suspensory ligament of ovary, broad ligament

Trans-abdominal ultrasound of ovary, longitudinal view

Developing ovarian follicles may be demonstrated with ultrasound as well defined anechoic areas usually in the periphery of the ovary; the appearances of which vary significantly throughout the menstrual cycle. The ovaries lie posteriorly in the pelvis, on either side of the uterus although their position can vary. Postero-lateral to the ovaries run the internal iliac vessels.

The gonadal arteries arise directly from the aorta in both males and females.

The ovary has three ligamentous attachments; the ovarian ligament connects the ovary to the uterus in the midline, the suspensory ligament of the ovary elevates the ovary towards the lateral pelvic wall and contains the ovarian vessels, lymphatics and nerves, while the broad ligament envelopes the ovaries, uterus and uterine (fallopian) tubes.

Q11 Answers

a Head of epididymis
b Rete testis
c Mediastinum testis

d Trace of fluid within tunica vaginalis/physiological hydrocele
e Vas deferens

Ultrasound of right testis, longitudinal view

The testis has a homogenous appearance on ultrasound. Several distinct structures are however identifiable.

An echogenic line running through the middle of the testis is known as the mediastinum testis and represents fibrous septae which divide the gland into lobules.

Within the superior end of the testis there is an area of increased echogenicity known as the rete testis. The rete testis is the confluence of the seminiferous tubules which convey sperm from the testis to the epididymis for storage and concentration.

A triangular-shaped area of similar echogenicity to the testis and lying immediately adjacent to its superior pole represents the head of the epididymis. The epididymis runs the length of the testis; at its distal end, the tail of the epididymis is continuous with the origin of the vas deferens. The vas deferens is the tube which delivers sperm from the testis to the ejaculatory duct in the prostatic urethra. From the distal end of the epididymis, the vas deferens turns 180 degrees and travels up the posterior wall of the scrotum. The vas deferens is often visible on ultrasound as a deeply situated tube running parallel to the testis and it becomes more prominent following vasectomy.

Q12 Answers

a Ischiocavernosus muscle
b Bulbospongiosus muscle
c Spermatic cord
d External anal sphincter
e The obturator externus is one of the external rotators of the hip

T1W MRI of male pelvic floor, axial slice

The penis is composed of three cylindrical bodies of erectile tissue, namely the corpus spongiosum (contains the urethra) and two paired corpora cavernosa (lie dorsally in the penis). In the pelvic floor the cavernosa divide to form the penile crura which lie along the ischiopubic rami, while the spongiosum forms the penile bulb in the midline. Muscular compression of these tissues by the ischiocavernosus and bulbospongiosus muscles at the root of the penis leads to erection.

The spermatic cord contains the structures running to and from the testis; the major structures include the vas deferens, testicular artery, pampiniform venous plexus and nerves.

The external anal sphincter is a ring of voluntary muscle surrounding the anal canal and is part of the levator ani muscle group.

Q13 Answers

a Iliacus muscle
b External iliac artery
c Opening of the prostatic urethra (internal urethral orifice)
d Obturator internus muscle
e Ligamentum teres of the hip

T2W MRI of male pelvis, coronal section through prostate

The prostate sits on the urogenital diaphragm in the lower pelvis immediately beneath the urinary bladder. The prostatic urethra can be visualised with MRI.

Iliacus is a hip flexor which arises from the iliac fossa (hence the name) and joins with the psoas major muscle in its attachment to the lesser trochanter of the femur. The obturator internus muscle is attached to the lateral wall of the pelvic cavity and leaves the pelvis posteriorly by passing through the lesser sciatic foramen to attach to the greater trochanter of the femur.

The external iliac artery runs along the medial border of psoas major before exiting the pelvis.

Q14 Answers

a Rectus abdominis muscle
b Urinary bladder
c Urethra surrounded by external urethral sphincter
d Vagina
e Levator ani muscle

T2W MRI of female pelvic floor, axial section

The female pelvic floor has many of the same constituents as the male equivalent. The urogenital diaphragm stretches between the two sides of the pubic arch and provides support for the vagina. In both sexes, the urethra passes through the urogenital diaphragm which forms the external urethral sphincter at this level.

The ischiocavernosus and bulbospongiosus muscles have a very similar location in both sexes (not shown here) but in females the bulbospongiosus surrounds the vagina and these muscles provide erectile function to the clitoris.

The levator ani are a group of muscles which close the pelvic outlet (pelvic diaphragm) and form a loop around the anus providing support at the level of the pelvic floor. Lateral to the levator ani muscles lie the ischioanal fossae. These are fat filled triangular spaces which normally accommodate rectal expansion when required. Occasionally the ischioanal fossae can become infected leading to an ischioanal abscess. An ischioanal abscess can spontaneously open into both the anal canal and perineal skin leading to the formation of a perianal fistula.

Q15 Answers

a Endometrium
b Junctional zone of myometrium
c Trace of fluid in the recto-uterine pouch (of Douglas)
d Endocervical canal
e Myometrium of uterus

T2W MRI of female pelvis, midline sagittal section

T2W MRI is often used to evaluate the uterus as its zonal anatomy can be appreciated. The endometrium, endocervical canal and vaginal canal all appear with high signal intensity. The myometrium is divided into the low signal, inner junctional zone and the intermediate signal of uterine bulk. Both the internal and external cervical os can usually be seen at either end of the endocervical canal. The cervix normally protrudes into the upper vagina creating anterior and posterior recesses, known as the fornices. The position of the uterus is readily appreciated relative to the bladder; the normal position is anteverted (angle between vagina and uterus) and anteflexed (angle between cervix and uterus) meaning it lies anterior to the cervix and curves anteriorly over the bladder (as shown).

The deepest intraperitoneal part of the female pelvis is the space between the posterior uterus and anterior rectum. This is known as the recto-uterine pouch (of Douglas) and will often be seen to contain a trace of free peritoneal fluid (as a consequence of ovulation). In pathological states, this area is also where free fluid may collect first.

Q16 Answers

a Seminal vesicle
b Perirectal/mesorectal fascia
c Perirectal and pararectal fat
d Natal cleft
e Coccygeus muscle

TIW MRI of male pelvis at level of seminal vesicles, axial section

The seminal vesicles produce the medium in which sperms are transmitted from the body. The seminal vesicles lie on either side of the midline posterior to the prostate and bladder and anterior to the rectum in males. T2W MRI shows the seminal vesicles to be fluid filled.

The rectum is surrounded by fat within which is a layer known as the perirectal (or mesorectal) fascia. The perirectal fascia is an important plane to identify when staging rectal cancer using MRI.

The coccygeus muscle extends from the inferior sacrum and coccyx to the ischial spine and is one of the muscles of the pelvic diaphragm along with the levator ani group. The pelvic diaphragm separates the pelvic cavity from the perineum.

Q17 Answers

a Sacroiliac joint
b Sacral nerve root in sacral foramina
c Obturator internus muscle
d Rectum
e Levator ani muscle

T1W MRI showing rectum and posterior pelvis, coronal section

The sacroiliac joints are synovial joints but have very little mobility. They are strong weight bearing joints which link the spine to the pelvis. On MRI, the sacroiliac joints should show the interlocking corticated edges of both the sacrum and ileum.

The sacral nerves enter the pelvic cavity through the anterior sacral foramina as is demonstrated on this image. Sacral nerves supply the pelvis and lower limb.

The obturator internus muscle is an external rotator of the hip and covers most of the lateral wall of the pelvic cavity.

Q18 Answers

a Urinary bladder
b Right seminal vesicle
c Central zone of the prostate
d Prostatic urethra
e Peripheral zone of prostate

T2W MRI of prostate, coronal section

The prostate usually measures 3–5cm in length and sits inferior to the urinary bladder. The first part of the urethra passes through the prostate and is therefore named the prostatic urethra. Both transrectal ultrasound and T2W MRI can demonstrate the peripheral, central and transitional zones of the prostate. Most of the glandular tissue of the prostate can be found in the peripheral zone. On coronal T2W MRI the peripheral zone is seen as a high signal 'U' shaped area surrounding the lower signal superiorly placed central zone. The transitional zone surrounds the midportion of the urethra (not well seen here) and is not always differentiated from the central zone. The 'central gland' is a term used to describe the central and transitional zones collectively. With increasing age the transitional zone tends to hypertrophy; this can lead to an increase in size of the central gland which may reduce the diameter of the prostatic urethra leading to urinary outflow problems.

The seminal vesicles sit on either side of the midline postero-superiorly to the prostate and are fluid filled.

Q19 Answers

a The aorta bifurcates into the right and left common iliac arteries at the level of L4
b Inferior mesenteric artery
c The internal iliac artery has anterior and posterior divisions
d Inferior epigastric artery or deep circumflex iliac artery
e The gonadal arteries (testicular or ovarian) arise directly from the abdominal aorta at the level of L2

Abdomino-pelvic MRA

The abdominal aorta is a direct continuation of the thoracic aorta and runs from the aortic opening in the diaphragm at T12 to its bifurcation into the two common iliac vessels at the level of L4. In the infra renal portion, the major branches are the right and left gonadal arteries, the inferior mesenteric artery and usually four paired lumbar arteries. The gonadal vascular and lymphatic vessels are in similar locations meaning lymph of testicular or ovarian origin will drain to para-aortic nodes.

The internal iliac artery supplies the pelvis; the posterior division has branches to the posterior pelvic wall and musculature while the anterior division supplies the pelvic viscera and perineum. The external iliac artery predominantly supplies the lower limb becoming the common femoral artery as it passes under the inguinal ligament. Just before leaving the pelvis however, the external iliac artery has two branches which supply the anterior abdominal wall, namely the inferior epigastric and the deep circumflex iliac arteries.

LOWER LIMB

Q1

a Name the muscle that attaches to the structure labelled A
b Name the ligament that attaches to the structure labelled A
c Name the line labelled C
d Name the structure labelled D
e Name the structure labelled E

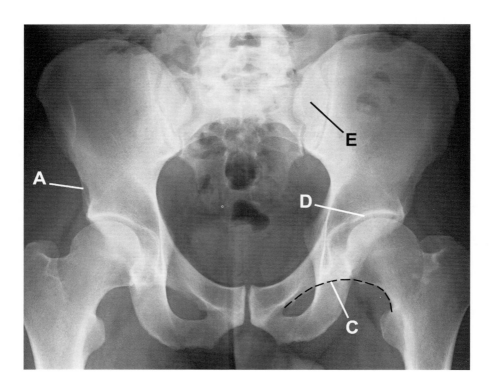

Q2

a Name the structure labelled A
b Name the structure labelled B
c Name the structure labelled C
d Name the angle labelled D
e Name the structure labelled E

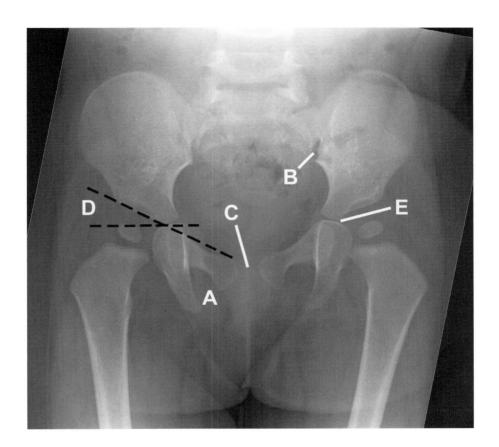

Q3

a Name the structure labelled A
b Name the structure labelled B
c Name the structure labelled C
d Name the structure labelled D
e Name the structure labelled E

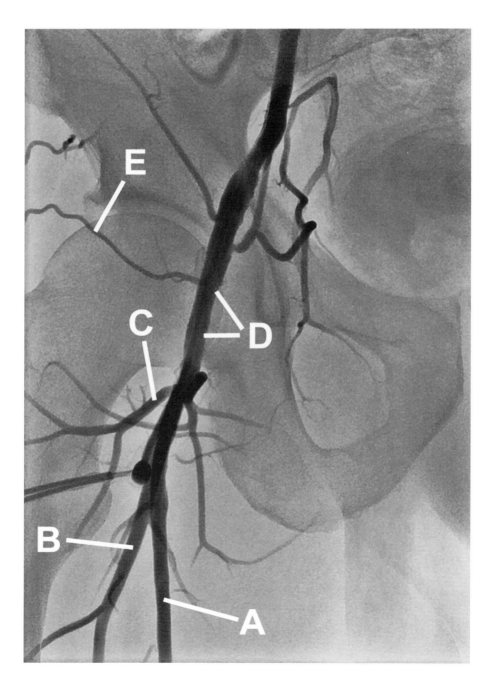

Q4

a Name the structure labelled A
b Name the angle labelled B
c Name the angle labelled C
d Name the structure labelled D
e Name the structure labelled E

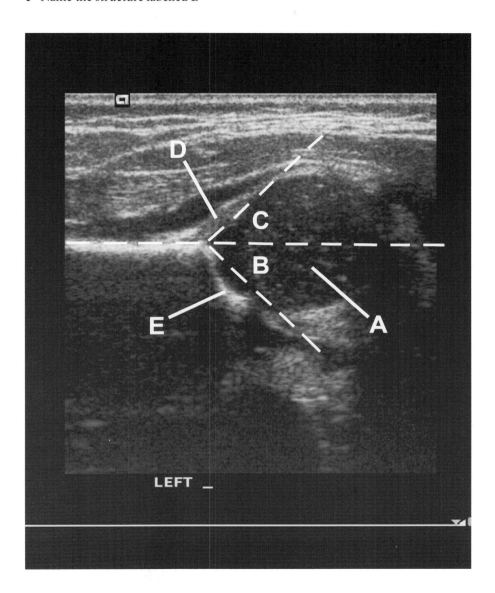

Q5

a Name the structure labelled A
b Name the structure labelled B
c Name the structure positioned lateral to structure A
d Name the space immediately medial to structure A
e Name the major superficial vein which drains into structure A

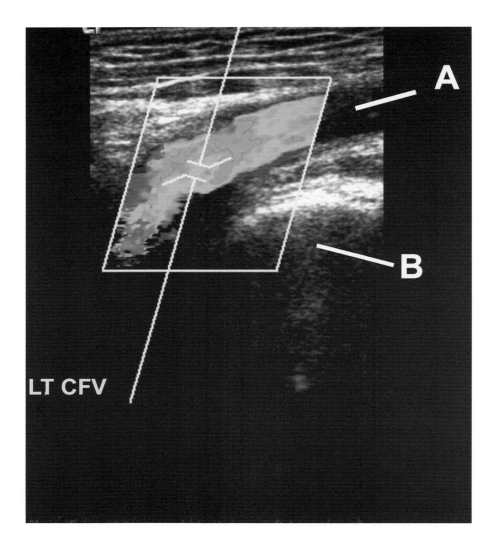

Q6

a Name the nerve labelled A
b Name the nerve labelled B
c Name the structure labelled C
d Name the structure labelled D
e Name the structure labelled E

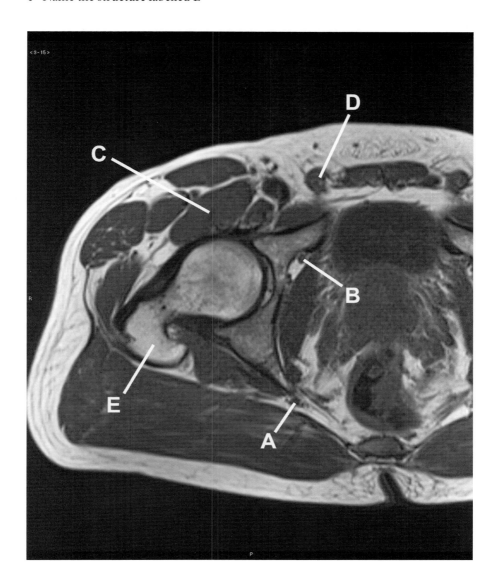

Q7

a Name the structure labelled A
b Name the structure labelled B
c Name the structure labelled C
d Name the structure labelled D
e Name the structure labelled E

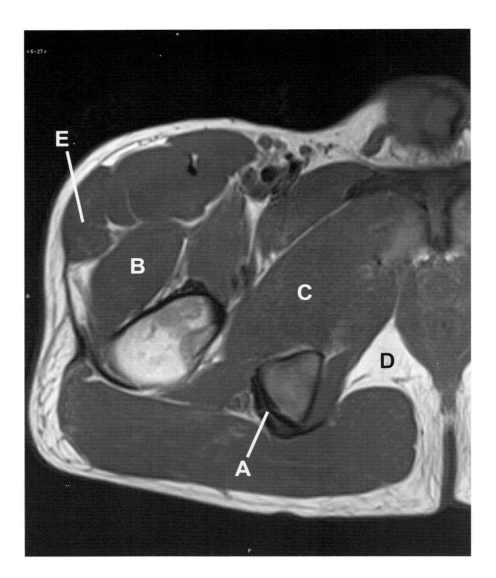

Q8

a Name the structure labelled A
b Name the structure labelled B
c Name the structure that runs through the groove labelled C
d Name the structure labelled D
e Name the structure labelled E

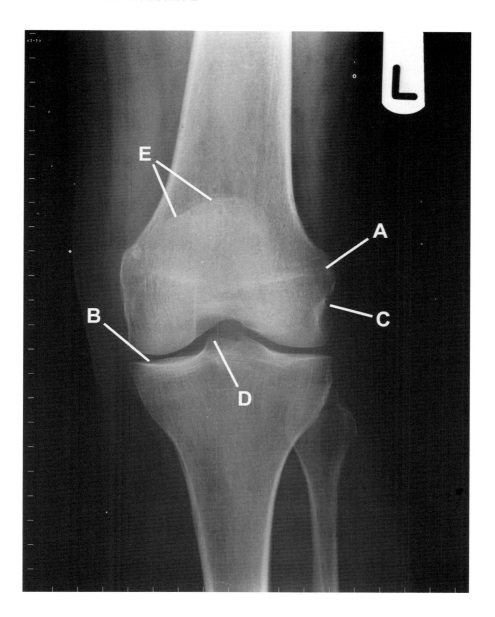

Q9

a Name the structure labelled A
b Name the structure labelled B
c Name the structure labelled C
d Name the structure labelled D
e Define the age at which ossification of the patella normally begins

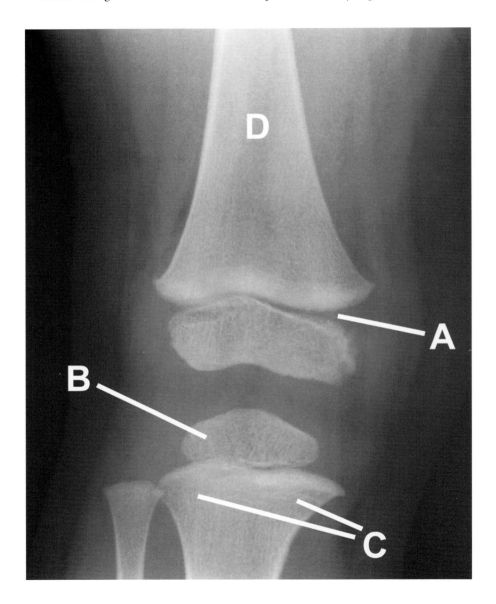

Q10

a Name the structure labelled A
b Name the structure labelled B
c Name the structure labelled C
d Name the structure labelled D
e Name the structure labelled E

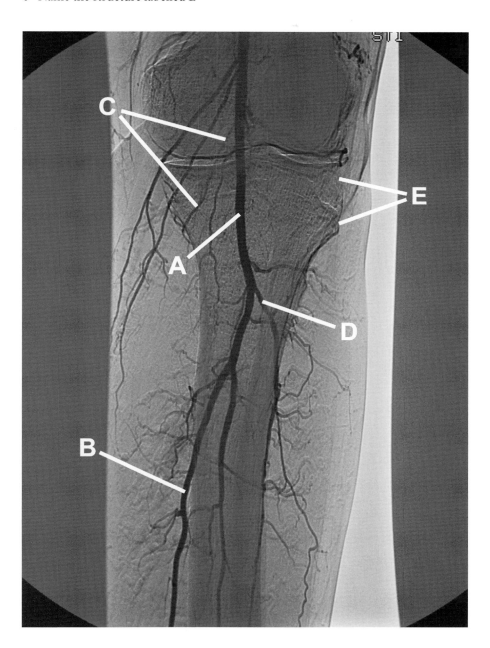

Q11

a Name the structure labelled A
b Name the structure labelled B
c Name the structure labelled C
d Name the structure labelled D
e Name the structure labelled E

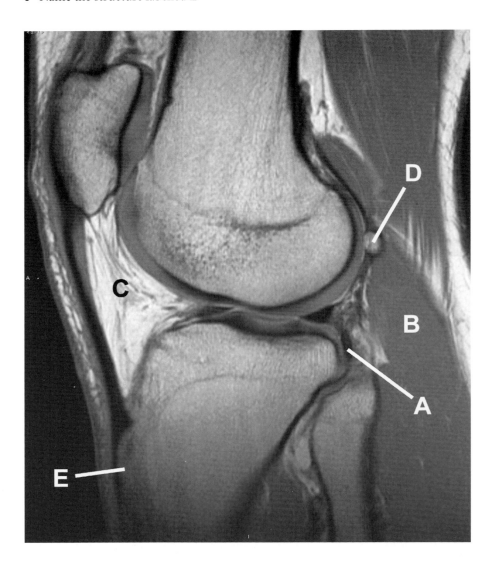

Q12

a Name the structure labelled A
b Name the structure labelled B
c Name the structure labelled C
d Name the structure labelled D
e Name the structure labelled E

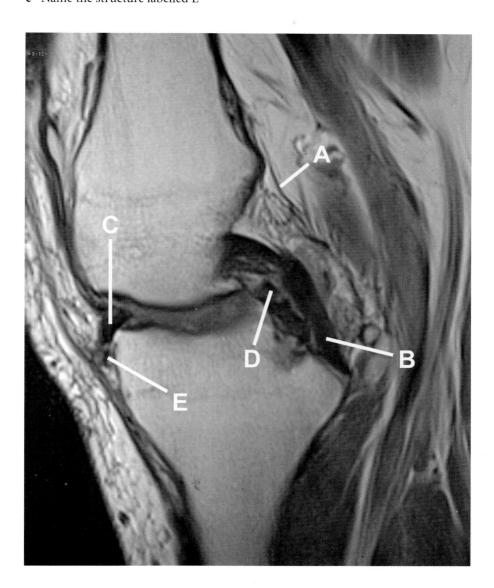

Q13

a Name the structure labelled A
b Name the structure labelled B
c Name the structure labelled C
d Name the structure labelled D
e Name the structure labelled E

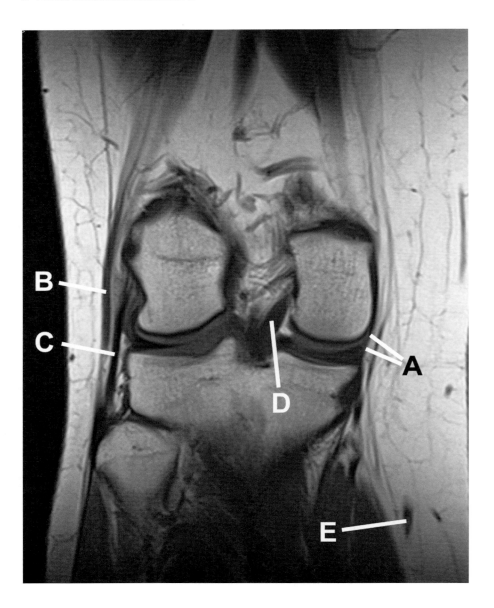

Q14

a Name the structure labelled A
b Name the structure labelled B
c Name the structure labelled C
d Name the structure labelled D
e Name the structures labelled E

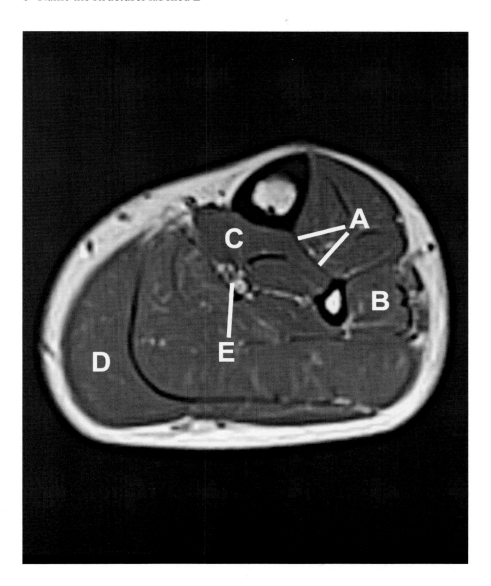

Q15

a Name the structure labelled A
b Name the structure labelled B
c Name the joint space labelled C
d Name the structure labelled D
e Define the normal angle at the position labelled E

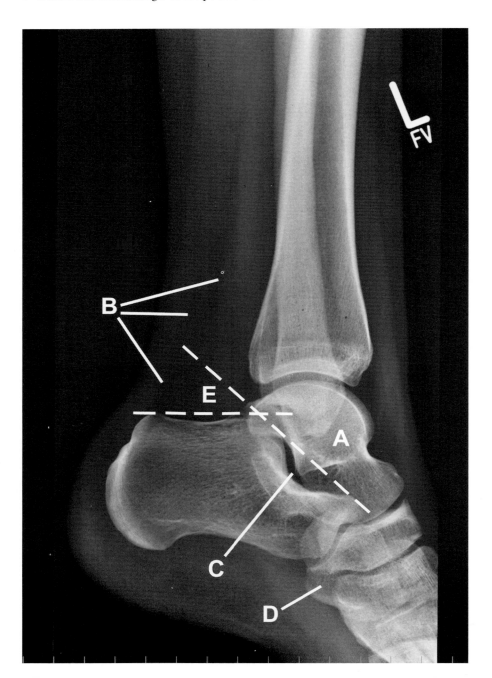

Q16

a Name the structure labelled A
b Name the structure labelled B
c Name the structure labelled C
d Name the structure labelled D
e Name the structure labelled E

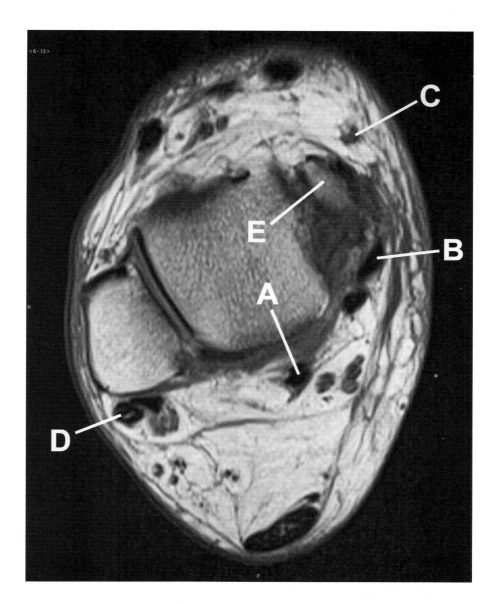

Q17

a Name the structure labelled A
b Name the structure labelled B
c Name the structure labelled C
d Name the structure labelled D
e Name the structure labelled E

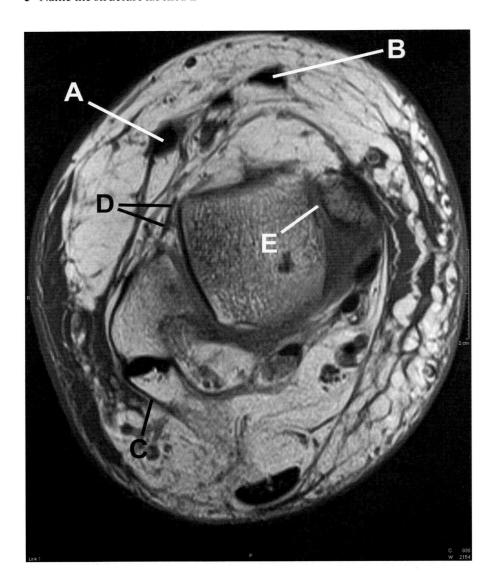

Q18

a Name the structure labelled A
b Name the structure labelled B
c Name the structure labelled C
d Name the structure labelled D
e Name the structure labelled E

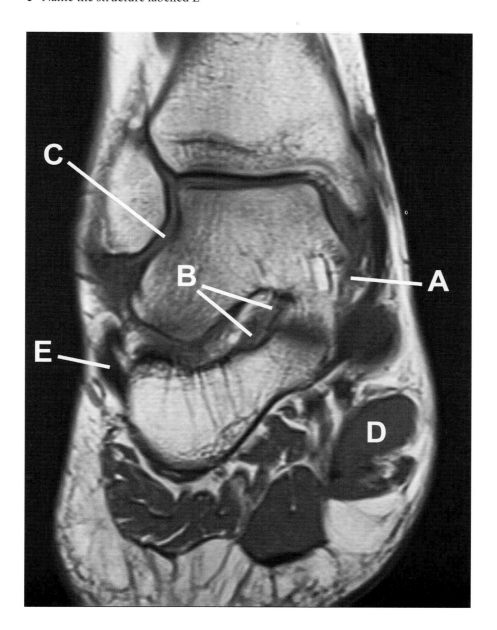

Q19

a Name the structure labelled A
b Name the structure labelled B
c Name the structure labelled C
d Name the level of the spinal nerve root supplying structure D
e Name the structure labelled E

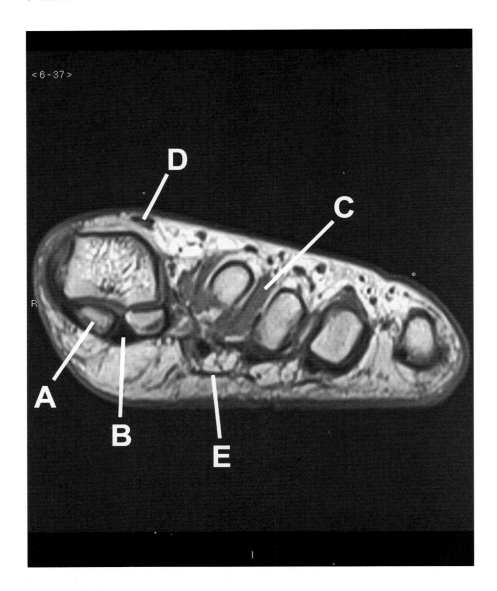

Q20

a Name the structure labelled A
b Name the structure labelled B
c Name the structure labelled C
d Name the sensory dermatome at the site labelled D
e Name the structure labelled E

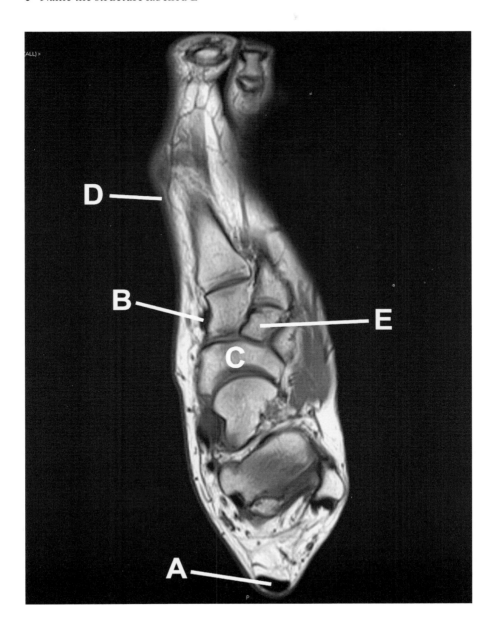

6

LOWER LIMB – ANSWERS

Q1 Answers

a Straight head of rectus femoris muscle
b Iliofemoral ligament (of Bigelow)
c Shenton's line
d Acetabular roof
e Sacral ala

Radiograph of pelvis, AP view

A number of lower limb muscles originate from the bony pelvis. Of the anterior femoral muscles, sartorius and tensor fascia lata originate from the anterior superior iliac spine (ASIS) while the straight head of rectus femoris arises from the anterior inferior iliac spine (AIIS). The adductor muscles including gracillis and pectineus arise from the pubic bone. The largest of these, adductor magnus, also takes origin from the ischiopubic ramus and the ischial tuberosity. The three hamstrings also arise from the ischial tuberosity. The ASIS and AIIS both have accessory ossification centres which appear at puberty and fuse at around 25 years.

The hip joint is stabilized by three ligaments and the joint capsule. The capsule encloses the femoral head and neck and is strongest in the anterior and superior portions. The iliofemoral ligament (of Bigelow) attaches the ASIS to the intertrochanteric line. Posterior support is provided by the ischiofemoral ligament and inferior support by the pubofemoral ligament.

Shenton's line should course a smooth, unbroken curve along the underside of the femoral neck, acetabulum and superior pubic ramus on an AP pelvic radiograph. This was originally described specifically in relation to tuberculosis of the hip, however a variety of hip conditions can cause interruption or angulation of this line. When assessing the posterior (ilioischial) and anterior (iliopubic) columns of the acetabulum with a radiograph, oblique projections (Judet views) are commonly used.

The sacral ala is the wing-like portion positioned lateral to the sacral body which is the product of fused costal elements and transverse processes of the sacral vertebrae.

Shenton EWH. Disease in bone and its detection by the X-Rays. 1911; *Macmillan*:42–43.

Q2 Answers

a Ischiopubic synchondrosis
b Sacroiliac joint
c Symphysis pubis
d Acetabular angle
e Triradiate cartilage of the acetabulum

Pelvic radiograph in a 12 month-old infant, AP view

The inonimate bones of the pelvis are made up of the ilium, ischium and pubis. In infants and children these bones are each separated by a radiolucent physis. The three bones converge at the triradiate cartilage of the acetabulum.

Assessment of the acetabulum and femoral head on paediatric radiographs can be complemented using two principal measurements. Both of these utilize a line drawn connecting the tri-radiate cartilages on both sides (known as the 'Y–Y' or Hilgenreiner line).

The acetabular angle is measured between the Y–Y line and a line along the ossified acetabular concavity and pubic ramus. This angle is approximately 28 degrees at birth and decreases gradually with age, reflecting normal bony maturation of the acetabulum. Developmental dysplasia of the hip (DDH) often results in an increased acetabular angle.

Positioning of the femoral head can be assessed by adding a line which is drawn perpendicular to the Hilgenreiner line at the outer acetabular margin (known as the Perkins line). These will serve to divide the hip into quadrants. The normal location of the ossified femoral head is in the infero-medial quadrant.

The sacro-iliac joints are synovial joints but despite this have very little movement. They are extensively reinforced by means of the anterior, posterior and interosseous sacroiliac ligaments. The pubic symphisis is a secondary cartilaginous joint which is normally immobile.

Norton KI, Polin SAM. Developmental Dysplasia of the Hip. *Radiology* 2009; eMedicine: www.emedicine.medscape.com

Q3 Answers

a Superficial femoral artery
b Profunda femoris artery
c Lateral circumflex femoral artery
d Common femoral artery
e Superficial circumflex iliac artery

Digital subtraction angiogram right groin

The external iliac artery becomes the common femoral artery after passing beneath the inguinal ligament, midway between the ASIS and pubic tubercle. Four arteries take their origin from the proximal common femoral artery. The superficial circumflex iliac arteries course laterally towards the femoral neck and ASIS. Running in a medial direction are the superficial epigastric artery and the superficial and deep (external) pudendal arteries.

The circumflex arteries contribute to an anastomosis with the inferior gluteal artery which encircles the proximal femur, providing most of its blood supply. Branches from this anastomosis enter the outer hip capsule to supply the femoral neck. An additional blood supply comes through the ligamentum teres, though this is minimal in the fully developed hip making the femoral head susceptible to avascular necrosis following intracapsular proximal femoral fractures. The descending branch of the lateral femoral circumflex artery also forms an anastomosis with the geniculate arteries around the knee and this can provide a path of collateralization to the leg in cases of superficial femoral artery occlusion.

The common femoral artery divides into the superficial femoral artery and profunda femoris artery, the latter of which principally supplies the thigh.

Q4 Answers

a Femoral head
b Alpha angle
c Beta angle
d Cartilaginous acetabular roof
e Osseus acetabular concavity

Hip ultrasound in a 6 month-old child, coronal view

Normal development of the hip joint is reliant on there being adequate contact between the femoral head and acetabulum. Abnormalities of subluxation and dislocation need to be recognized in order to prevent dysplastic development. In infants there is a discrepancy in size between the large femoral head and the relatively under developed acetabulum and since the hip joint is predominantly cartilaginous, the preferred modality for assessment is ultrasound.

The ilium, ossified acetabulum and cartilaginous acetabulum are all seen on coronal imaging. The non-ossified femoral head has a 'speckled' echotexture. There are three lines which enable assessment of the hip joint: the 'baseline' runs parallel to the ilium; the 'acetabular roofline' runs along the plane of the bony acetabular concavity and the 'inclination' line runs from the lateral bony acetabulum along the underside of the cartilaginous roof.

The alpha angle is a measurement of acetabular depth (and therefore maturity) and lies between the baseline and acetabular roofline. The beta angle is a measurement of acetabular cartilaginous roof coverage and lies between the baseline and the inclination line. Dysplastic hips have a low alpha angle and high beta angle (i.e. immature bony acetabulum and predominantly cartilaginous coverage of the femoral head). An alpha angle >60 degrees and beta angle <55 degrees is normal.

An alternative assessment of acetabular maturity is to define the distance from the medial aspect of the femoral head to the baseline as a percentage of total femoral head diameter. This is known as the d/D ratio and a value >58% is considered normal.

Norton KI, Polin SAM. Developmental Dysplasia of the Hip. *Radiology* 2009; eMedicine: www. emedicine.medscape.com

Q5 Answers

a Common femoral vein (CFV)
b Femoral head
c Femoral artery
d Femoral canal
e Long saphenous vein

Colour flow Doppler of the common femoral vein, longitudinal view

The walls of veins, like arteries, comprise of three layers; the endothelium-lined tunica intima, muscular tunica media and the connective tissue covering of tunica adventitia. Where the wall architecture of arteries and veins differ is in the thickness of these three layers and of the muscular medial layer in particular. This is relatively thin in the walls of veins which results in them being unable to oppose radial compression – a feature that can help distinguish between artery and vein on ultrasound examination. Lateral to the femoral vein lies the femoral artery. The femoral canal lies medial to the femoral vein and usually contains a lymph node (of Cloquet).

The hip joint lies deep to the common femoral vessels. As the femoral vein passes beyond the superior margin of the femoral head it adopts a deeper course before passing beneath the inguinal ligament and becoming the external iliac vein. The femoral head is used as a radiological landmark in percutaneous femoral arterial punctures to ensure that the arteriotomy is inferior to the inguinal ligament and therefore controllable with manual compression on the groin.

Q6 Answers

a Sciatic nerve
b Obturator nerve
c Iliopsoas muscle
d Spermatic cord
e Greater trochanter of the femur

T1W MRI hip and pelvis, axial section

The sciatic nerve (spinal nerves L4, 5, S1, 2, 3) is the largest nerve to emerge from the sacral plexus and exits the pelvis through the greater sciatic foramen to lie within the buttock. As it travels inferiorly in the posterior compartment of the thigh, branches emerge to supply the hamstring muscles. At the level of the upper popliteal fossa, it divides into the tibial and common peroneal nerves. The tibial nerve remains in the posterior compartment of the leg and supplies the flexor muscles of the calf. The common peroneal nerve swings laterally around the neck of the fibula where it divides into a superficial branch supplying the lateral compartment (evertors) and a deep branch supplying the anterior compartment (extensors) in the leg. Damage to the sciatic nerve can therefore have a devastating effect on lower limb function.

The obturator and femoral nerves are branches from the lumbar plexus (L2, 3, 4) and supply the obturator/adductor and the anterior thigh muscles respectively. Both nerves also supply sensory branches to the skin as well as the hip and knee joints. The femoral nerve exits the pelvis lateral to the artery in the femoral triangle. Medial to the femoral artery is the femoral vein, medial to which is the fat filled femoral canal. The obturator nerve exits through the obturator foramen which is located in the lateral wall of the pelvis adjacent to the common iliac bifurcation. The spermatic cord passes through the inguinal canal which is superficial and superior to the femoral canal and runs in a medial direction. All three of these channels – the femoral canal, the obturator foramen and the inguinal canal – are common sites of intestinal herniation.

Iliopsoas is the joining of the psoas major and iliacus muscles which forms at the inner aspect of the ilium. It runs anteriorly to pass beneath the inguinal ligament before inserting into the lesser trochanter of the femur.

Q7 Answers

a Common tendinous origin of the hamstrings
b Vastus lateralis
c Adductor magnus
d Ischio-anal fossa
e Tensor fascia lata

T1W MRI at greater trochanter level, axial section

The anterior femoral muscles comprise of the iliopsoas, tensor fascia lata, sartorius and quadriceps muscles. Tensor fascia lata arises from the ASIS and inserts into the iliotibial tract which is a strong band of fascia on the lateral aspect of the thigh (fascia lata). This inserts into the fibular head. Sartorius is a narrow muscle which also originates from the ASIS and courses superficially across the thigh to insert into the medial tibial condyle. The quadriceps is made up of the three vastus muscles (lateralis, medialis and intermedius) and rectus femoris. These all share a common tendinous insertion into the tibial tuberosity via the patellar tendon and serve to extend the knee joint. Rectus femoris arises from the AIIS and the acetabulum, vastus lateralis and medialis from the greater trochanter and the linea aspera and vastus intermedius from the anterior femoral shaft. All four quadriceps muscles are supplied by the femoral nerve (L3, 4).

The hamstrings (semimembranosus, semitendinosus and biceps femoris) share a common tendinous origin from the ischial tuberosity. Biceps femoris attaches to the fibular head while semimembranosus and semitendinosus insert into the medial tibia. All are supplied by the profunda femoris artery and the sciatic nerve.

The adductor muscles are separated from the anterior thigh muscles by the medial intermuscular septum, which attaches to the fascia lata. There is no septum dividing them from the posterior compartment. They consist of gracilis and the three adductors: longus, brevis and magnus. All take origin from the pubis, with magnus having a second origin alongside the hamstrings from the ischial tuberosity. Gracilis crosses the inner aspect of the thigh superficially to insert into the superior medial tibia behind sartorius. The adductors insert into the linea aspera of the femur and in the case of adductor magnus, also into the adductor tubercle. These muscles are supplied by the obturator nerve and by the profunda femoris and obturator arteries.

The ischio-anal (also known as ischio-rectal) fossae lie below and lateral to the levator ani muscles and are enclosed by the sacrotuberous ligaments and gluteus maximus posteriorly, obturator internus fascia laterally and the urogenital perineum inferiorly. Within these fatty spaces run the pudendal vessels and nerves. They are significant as a potential site of abscess formation, which can complicate sepsis of the rectum or anal canal.

Q8 Answers

a Lateral femoral epicondyle
b Medial tibial plateau
c Popliteus tendon
d Medial tibial spine or tubercle of intercondylar eminence
e Patella

AP radiograph of knee

The tibiofemoral space should normally measure 3–8mm. The tibial plateaus match the shape of the respective femoral condyles with the medial side being smaller and more rounded. The tibial spines, or tubercles of the intercondylar eminence, are the distal attachment of both anterior and posterior cruciate ligaments (ACL and PCL, respectively).

Popliteus is the only muscle that enters the knee joint.

Q9 Answers

a Distal femoral epiphyseal (growth) plate
b Proximal tibial epiphysis
c Proximal tibial metaphysis
d Femoral diaphysis
e 3–6 years

AP knee radiograph in a 2 year-old child

Long bone formation and growth occur as a result of cartilaginous ossification. All long bones have a cartilaginous growth plate or epiphyseal plate. The ossified bone on either side of this is known as the epiphysis (distal) and metaphysis (proximal). The shaft of a long bone is the diaphysis and the junction between it and the metaphysis is termed the diametaphysis. An apophysis is an ossified area which is located on one side of the bone. Apophyses do not normally contribute to increasing the length of a bone and are usually situated at the site of a tendinous insertion, for example at the 5th metatarsal base.

Ossification of the patella begins sometime between the ages of three and six and is usually completed by the onset of puberty. Ossification originates in several different locations that normally coalesce to form a single bone. Occasionally one centre (typically the upper lateral quadrant) will not fuse with the others which results in a bipartite patella.

Q10 Answers

a Popliteal artery
b Posterior tibial artery

c Medial genicular artery
d Anterior tibial artery
e Fibular head

Digital subtraction angiogram of leg, AP view

The popliteal artery is a continuation of the superficial femoral artery. It gives off seven branches within the popliteal fossa which supply the knee joint and adjacent muscles: superior/inferior muscular branches; medial superior/inferior geniculatar branches; lateral superior/inferior geniculatar branches and the middle genicular branch.

The popliteal artery divides into the anterior tibial artery and posterior tibial artery below the knee. Just distal to this division, the peroneal artery branches from the posterior tibial artery (as seen on this image). As these three branches diverge within a short distance, this area is often referred to as the popliteal trifurcation.

Q11 Answers

a Popliteus tendon
b Lateral head of gastrocnemius
c Infrapatellar (Hoffa's) fat pad
d Fabella
e Tibial tuberosity

T1W MRI knee, lateral sagittal section

A spherical osseous or cartilaginous fabella (Latin for 'little bean'), is occasionally seen in the vicinity of the knee. The location can be variable though it is usually within the lateral head of gastrocnemius muscle, in the postero-lateral aspect of the knee.

The popliteus muscle has its inferior origin above the soleal line of the posterior tibia. It runs in a supero-lateral course to its tendinous insertion into the groove on the lateral femoral condyle. Further insertion sites are at the posterior fibular head and the posterior lateral meniscus and these act to buttress the postero-lateral aspect of the knee joint. The action of popliteus is as the primary internal rotator of the tibia on the femur and it is the only muscle to enter the knee joint capsule. It also acts to laterally rotate the femur on the fixed tibia effectively unlocking the knee to allow flexion of the extended knee.

The joint capsule contains a triangular, anterior fat-pad sitting deep to the patellar tendon and surrounded by synovium. This is the infrapatellar (Hoffa's) fat pad which contains the deep infra-patellar bursa within its inferior aspect.

The tibial tuberosity is the bony ridge on the anterior tibial border into which the quadriceps tendon inserts.

Seebacher JR, Inglis AE, Marshall JL, Warren RF. The Structure of the Posterolateral Aspect of the Knee. *J Bone Joint Surg [Am]* 1982; 64:536–541.

Q12 Answers

a Posterior knee joint capsule
b Posterior cruciate ligament
c Anterior horn of lateral meniscus
d Anterior meniscofemoral ligament (of Humphrey)
e Transverse ligament

TIW MRI of knee, oblique sagittal section

The cruciate ligaments lie entirely within the knee joint capsule and are principally involved in the provision of antero-posterior joint stability. They both achieve this by adjoining the side of the tibial intercondylar process to its contralateral femoral condyle and are named according to the location of their tibial insertions. The PCL passes upwards, forwards and medially from the lateral aspect of the posterior tibial spine to the lateral aspect of the medial condyle. The ACL passes upwards, backwards and laterally from the anterior aspect of the tibial spine to the medial aspect of the lateral condyle.

The menisci consist of two semi-lunar fibrocartilages which serve to deepen the tibial articular surface. The medial meniscus is the larger of the two and, unlike the lateral meniscus, is attached firmly to its respective collateral ligament.

The appearance of meniscal ligaments can mimic meniscal pathology if incorrectly identified. The posterior horn of the lateral meniscus is attached to the medial femoral condyle by means of a meniscofemoral ligament which frequently splits into two parts to pass around the PCL. If the dominant part passes anterior to the PCL then it is known as the ligament of Humphrey, and if it passes posterior it is the ligament of Wrisberg. Anterior meniscal horns are interconnected by the transverse ligament.

Q13 Answers

a Medial collateral ligament
b Tendon of biceps femoris
c Lateral collateral ligament
d Posterior cruciate ligament
e Long saphenous vein

TIW MRI of knee, coronal section

The medial collateral ligament is a band-like structure which connects the medial femoral epicondyle to the tibial condyle. The lateral collateral ligament, which is more cord like, connects the lateral femoral epicondyle to the head of the fibula and is separated from the lateral joint capsule by the tendon of popliteus muscle. Additional lateral stability is provided via the ilio-tibial tract and biceps femoris, which share a common (conjoint) tendinous insertion into the postero-lateral fibular head. The other name for this insertion is the arcuate ligament. The tendon of popliteus passes under this on its way to its attachment to the lateral aspect of the lateral condyle of the femur.

The long saphenous vein (also known as the great saphenous vein) runs up the medial aspect of the leg and thigh to drain into the femoral vein at the sapheno-femoral junction. The short saphenous vein arises from the lateral aspect of the dorsal venous arch and passes posterior to the lateral malleolus. It runs up the back of the calf to drain into the popliteal vein at the sapheno-popliteal junction. The short and long saphenous veins are the two main superficial venous channels in the leg.

Q14 Answers

a Interosseous membrane
b Peroneus longus
c Tibialis posterior
d Medial head of gastrocnemius
e Posterior tibial neurovascular bundle

T1W MRI mid leg, axial section

Muscles of the leg are contained within three compartments: anterior (extensor); lateral (peroneal/evertor); and posterior (calf/flexor).

The anterior compartment contains the extensor muscles (tibialis anterior – TA, extensor hallucis longus – EHL, extensor digitorum longus – EDL and peroneus tertius) as well as the deep peroneal nerve and anterior tibial artery. It is bounded by the deep fascia and interosseous membrane and is a rigid compartment with limited scope for expansion.

The lateral compartment contains peroneus longus (PL) and peroneus brevis (PB) muscles plus the superficial peroneal nerve.

The posterior compartment is the largest and consists of superficial and deep groups which are divided by the deep transverse fascia. Soleus, the two heads of gastrocnemius and plantaris make up the superficial group whilst flexor digitorum longus (FDL), flexor hallucis longus (FHL) and tibialis posterior (TP) are the deep group. Also passing through this compartment are the posterior tibial and peroneal arteries and the tibial nerve.

Q15 Answers

a Talus
b Achilles tendon
c Posterior subtalar joint (talocalcaneal joint)
d Cuboid
e 30 degrees

Radiograph of ankle, lateral view

The talus consists of a head, neck and body and is a bone with no muscular attachments. As the name suggests, the neck is the slightly narrowed part of the talus which joins the body (posterior) and head (anterior). In adults it is angled such that it points roughly along the line of the first metatarsal.

The subtalar joint is functionally a single joint between the talus and calcaneum however it is made up of two components. The talocalcaneal (posterior) joint is between the posterior facet on the underside of the talus and the adjacent facet that is located on the upper calcaneum. The talocalcaneonavicular joint adjoins the talar head, the antero-superior surface of the calcaneum and the posterior surface of the navicular together with the spring ligament.

Bohler's angle is a means of assessing the calcaneal profile height. The lines converge on the anterior end of the superior articular facet, with one line beginning at the posterior end of the same articular facet and the other beginning at the postero-superior calcaneal margin: 30 degrees is normal. Calcaneal fractures are usually due to excessive axial loading (often resulting from a fall or a road traffic accident) which can cause impaction and flattening of the posterior facet and a reduction in Bohler's angle. In the context of trauma, an angle <23 degrees is highly suggestive of a calcaneal fracture.

Isaacs J, Baba M, Szomer ZS. FA5: The Diagnostic Accuracy of Böhler's Angle in Fractures of the Calcaneus. *J Bone Joint Surg [Br] Proceedings* 2010; 92: 178.

Q16 Answers

a Flexor hallucis longus tendon
b Tibialis posterior tendon
c Long saphenous vein
d Peroneus longus tendon
e Medial malleolus

T1W MRI of ankle, axial section

Tibialis posterior, flexor digitorum longus and flexor hallucis longus are three of the seven muscles of the posterior compartment of the leg (the remainder being gastrocnemius, soleus, popliteus and plantaris). All three take their origin from the middle third of the posterior tibia and/or fibula and insert onto the plantar aspect of the foot via long slender tendons that converge to pass behind the medial malleolus. Identifying which tendon is which is helped with the mnemonic 'Tom, Dick and Harry' (from medial to lateral the order in which they lie is **TP**, **FDL** and then F**HL**.)

The lateral (or peroneal) compartment contains the two peroneal muscles – longus and brevis. Peroneus longus tendon is the more superficial of the two above the ankle. Both muscles originate from the lateral aspect of the fibula and pass posterior to the lateral malleolus and beneath the peroneal retinaculum before inserting onto the 5th metacarpal (brevis) and medial cuneiform/1st metatarsal (longus). Insertion of the peroneus brevis tendon into the base of the 5th metatarsal renders this site susceptible to fracture in the context of ankle trauma. Despite its name, peroneus tertius is within the anterior compartment.

Q17 Answers

a Extensor digitorum tendon
b Tibialis anterior tendon
c Peroneal retinaculum
d Anterior inferior talofibular ligament
e Talotibial joint

T1W MRI of ankle, axial section

Tibialis anterior, extensor hallucis longus and extensor digitorum longus are three of the four anterior compartment muscles (the other being peroneus tertius) and originate from the anterior surface of the tibia and fibula. They form tendons above the ankle joint which pass anteriorly beneath the extensor retinaculum. Similar to their flexor counterparts their relative positions are constant in relation to each other at the ankle. Their configuration is slightly different however but this can be remembered using a variation on the mnemonic, which on this occasion is 'Tom, Harry and Dick' (from medial to lateral the order in which they lie is **TA**, **EHL** and then **EDL**).

Ligaments of the ankle joint are numerous and fall broadly into three groups:

1 The distal tibiofibular joint is classed as a syndesmosis and consists of anterior and posterior tibiofibular ligaments and the interosseous ligament which is a continuation of the interosseous membrane.
2 The medial (deltoid) ligament complex consists of (from anterior to posterior) the tibionavicular, tibiocalcaneal and posterior tibiotalar ligaments. The anterior portion of the deltoid ligament blends into the calcaneonavicular (or spring) ligament.
3 Three structures make up the lateral ligament complex and they are (from anterior to posterior) the anterior talofibular, calcaneofibular and posterior talofibular ligaments.

Q18 Answers

a Deep part of deltoid ligament
b Interosseous talocalcaneal ligament
c Talofibular joint
d Abductor hallucis muscle
e Peroneus longus tendon

T2W MRI of ankle, coronal section

This image demonstrates the anatomy of the lateral and medial (deltoid) collateral ligaments of the ankle and the subtalar (hindfoot) joint. The ankle joint permits dorsiflexion and plantarflexion of the foot. Mobility of the subtalar joint supplements this by enabling inversion (in plantarflexion) and eversion (in dorsiflexion) of the forefoot.

Three superficial first-layer plantar muscles arise from the calcaneus. Medial to lateral they are: abductor hallucis, flexor digitorum brevis (similar in function to its upper limb counterpart flexor digitorum superficialis), and abductor digiti minimi. All of these muscles are supplied via the S2 nerve root.

Q19 Answers

a Sesamoid bone
b Tendon of flexor hallucis longus
c Interosseous muscle
d L5
e Plantar aponeurosis

MRI of foot at distal metatarsal level, coronal section

Two sesamoid bones are normally seen on the plantar aspect of the foot where flexor hallucis brevis inserts to the 1st metatarsal head. Between them runs the tendon of flexor hallucis longus.

The muscles of the plantar aspect of the foot are divided in four layers, all of which lie deep to the plantar aponeurosis. They include the short flexors and abductors as well as the tendons of flexor digitorum longus and flexor hallucis longus. Interosseous muscles are arranged in a similar fashion as in the hands, comprising of plantar and dorsal layers which adduct and abduct the toes respectively (remember 'PAd' and 'DAb').

Extensor hallucis longus is supplied by the deep peroneal nerve and testing its function against resistance (e.g. standing on tip-toes) assesses the integrity of the anterior ramus of the L5 spinal nerve.

The plantar aponeurosis is a dense layer of collagen which extends across the sole of the foot. It arises from the medial side of the calcaneus to insert into the five metatarsophalyngeal joints and adds strength to the subcutaneous tissues of the sole.

Q20 Answers

a Achilles tendon
b Tendon of tibialis anterior muscle
c Navicular
d L4
e Intermediate cuneiform

T1W MRI of medial foot, axial section

The seven tarsal bones are arranged in three rows. The proximal row consists of the talus and calcaneus. Distally there are the three cuneiform bones (medial, intermediate and lateral) which are positioned medially and the cuboid which is positioned laterally. The middle row consists of the navicular which is on the medial side and lies between the talus and cuneiforms. On the lateral aspect of the foot the calcaneum articulates directly with the cuboid.

Several of the calf muscles insert onto the tarsal bones. Gastrocnemius and soleus, the large superficial muscles of the posterior calf, coalesce to form the Achilles tendon which attaches to the posterior surface of the calcaneum (plantaris is a small, slender vestigial calf muscle which sometimes contributes to this, but is absent in a number of people). Tibialis anterior has tendinous attachments to both the medial cuneiform and the base of the first metatarsal. Peroneus longus attaches to the same bones but on the inferior aspect. Tibialis posterior has many attachments: to the medial condyle of the navicular; to all of the tarsal bones (except the talus); and to the bases of the 2nd, 3rd and 4th metatarsals.

The dermatomes of the foot divide it into three regions positioned medial to lateral. The L4 dermatome includes the great toe. The L5 dermatome incorporates the central foot and 2nd to 4th toes, while the S1 dermatome includes the little toe and lateral foot.

Q1

a Name the structures labelled A
b Name the structure labelled B
c Name the structures labelled C
d Name the structure labelled D
e Name the structure labelled E

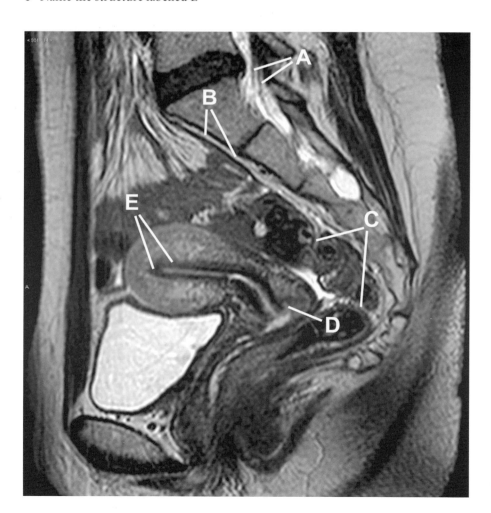

Q2

a Name the structure that attaches to A
b Name the structure labelled B
c Name the muscles contained within the anterior humeral compartment at the level indicated
d Name the structure labelled D
e Name the major ligaments that join the humerus to forearm bones

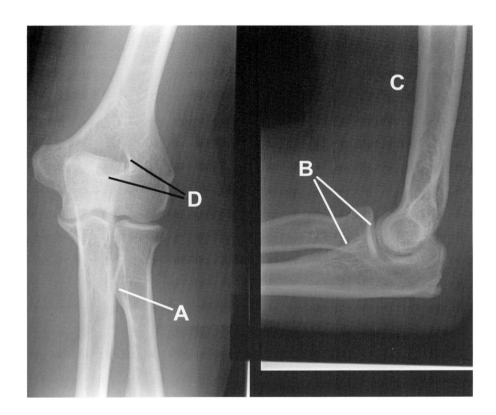

Q3

a Name the structure labelled A
b Name the structure labelled B
c Name the structure labelled C
d Name the structure labelled D
e Name the structure labelled E

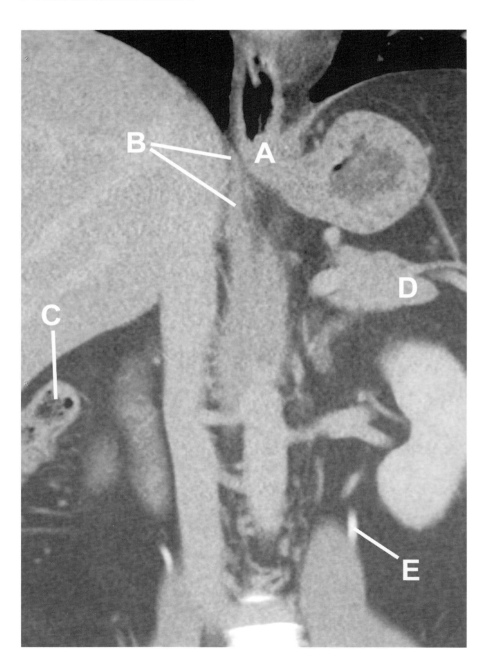

Q4

a Name the structure labelled A
b Name the structure labelled B
c Name the area labelled C
d Name the structure labelled D
e Name the anatomical variant demonstrated in this image

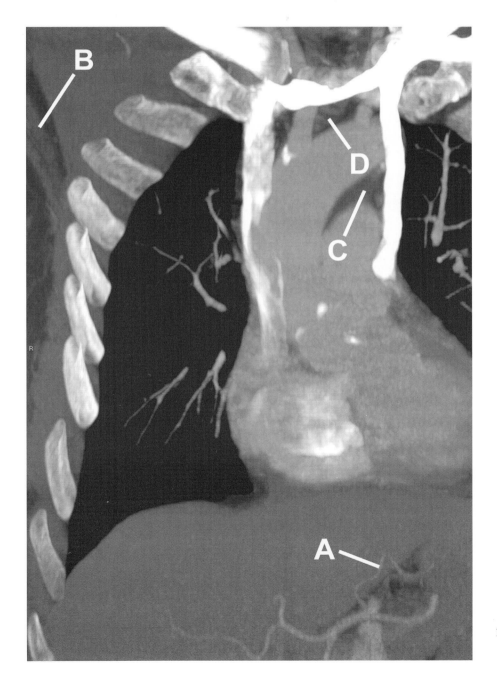

Q5

a Name the structure labelled A
b Name the structure labelled B
c Name the structure labelled C
d Name the structure labelled D
e Name the structure which separates the two lateral ventricles

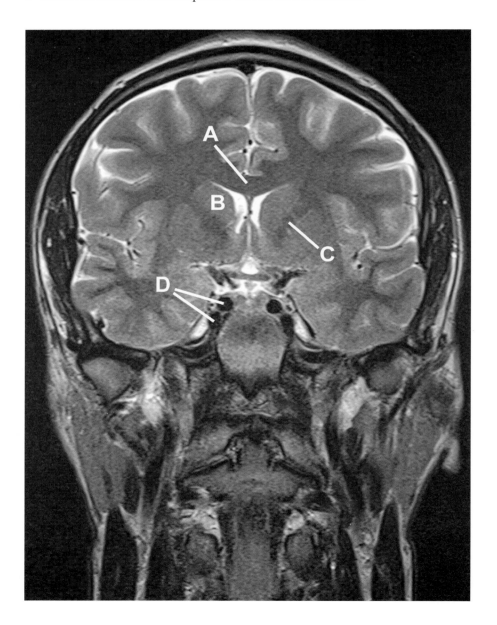

Q6

a Name the structure labelled A
b Name the structure labelled B
c Name the two lower limb muscles that attach to C
d Name the structure labelled D
e Name the structure labelled E

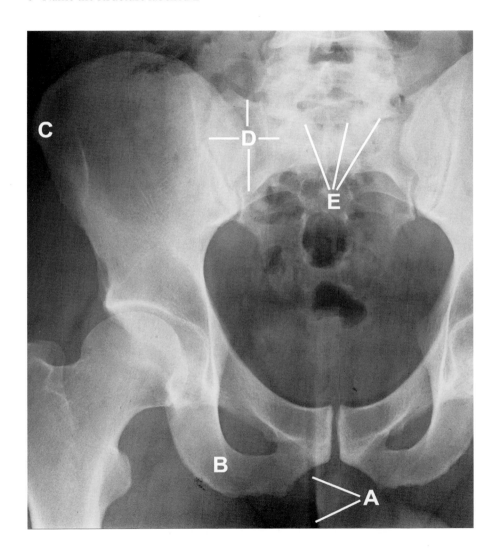

Q7

a Name the structure labelled A
b Name the space labelled B
c Name the part of the structure labelled C
d Name the structure labelled D
e Name the muscle that arises from both of the areas labelled E

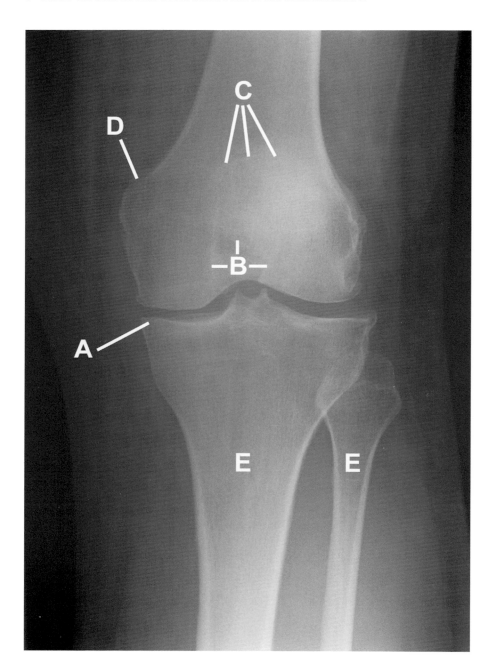

Q8

a   Name the structure labelled A
b   Name the structure labelled B
c   Name the structure labelled C
d   Name the structure labelled D
e   Name the structure labelled E

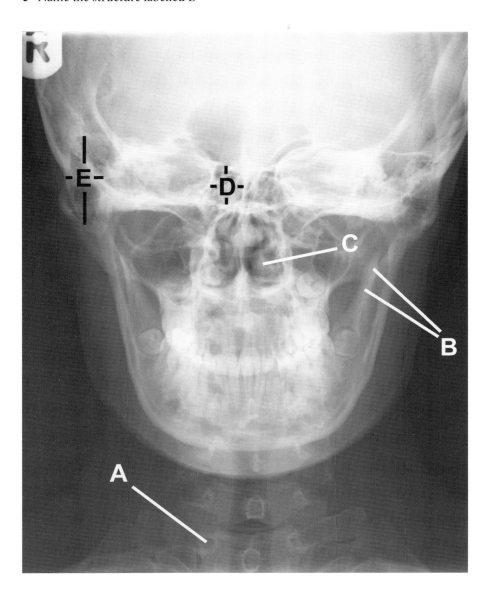

Q9

a Name the structure labelled A
b Name the structure that connects the two structures labelled B
c Name the structure labelled C
d Name the structure labelled D
e Name the structure labelled E

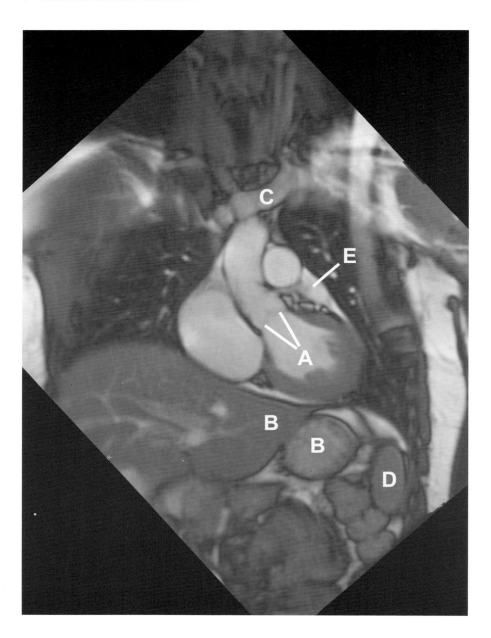

Q14

a Name the structure that links the radius and ulna in the space labelled A
b Name the structure labelled B
c Name the structure labelled C
d Name the structure labelled D
e Name the structures that the radial and ulnar arteries terminate as

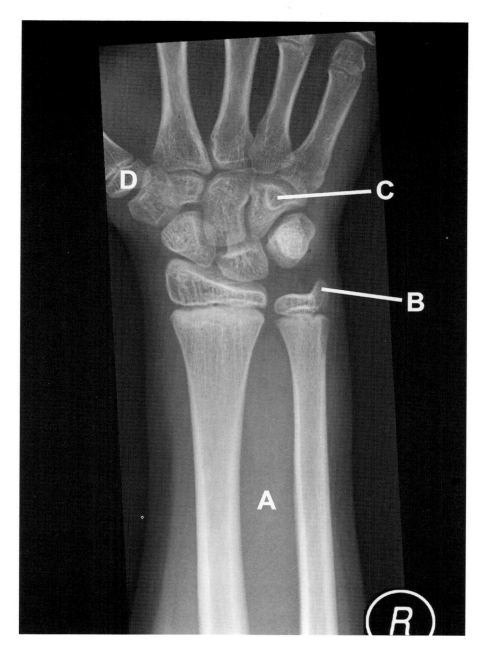

Q15

a Name the structures labelled A
b Name the structures labelled B
c Name the structure labelled C
d Name the structure labelled D
e Name the structures labelled E

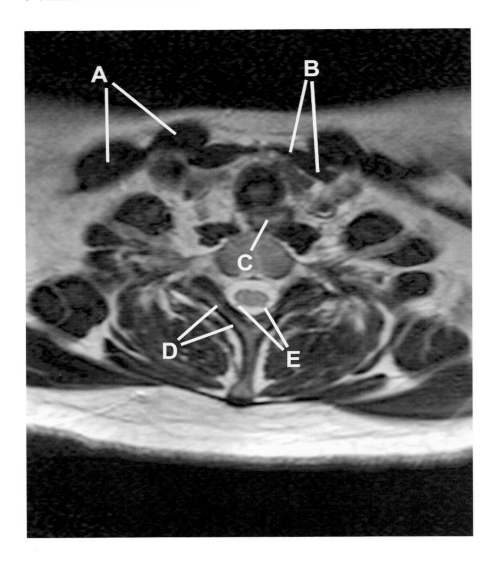

Q16

a Name the structure labelled A
b Name the structure labelled B
c Name the structure labelled C
d Name the structure labelled D
e Name the structure labelled E

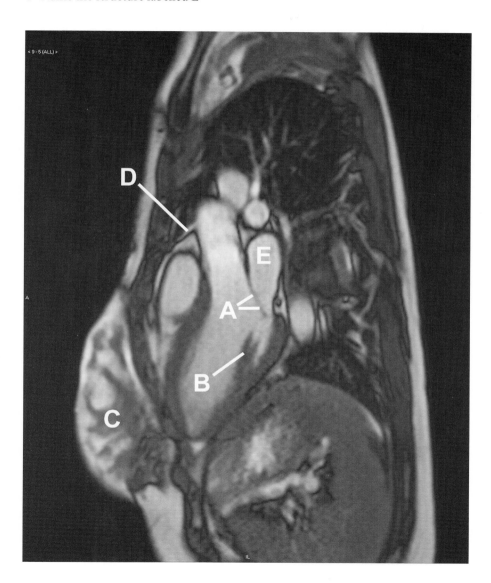

Q17

a Name the structure labelled A
b Name the structure labelled B
c Name the structure labelled C
d Name the structure labelled D
e Name the structure labelled E

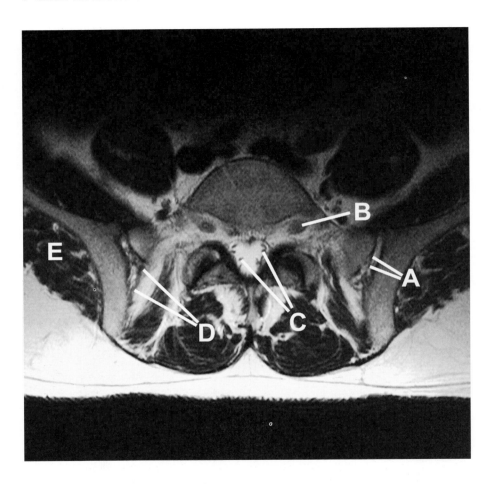

Q18

a Name the structure labelled A
b Name the structure labelled B
c Name the structure labelled C
d Name the structure labelled D
e Name the vertebral level at which the C5 spinal nerve exits the vertebral canal

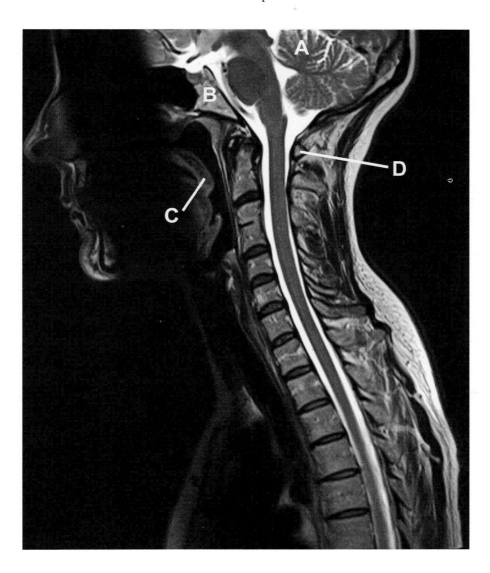

Q19

a Name the structure labelled A
b Name the group of neurovascular structures outlined and labelled B
c Name the structure labelled C
d Name the structure labelled D
e Name the structure labelled E

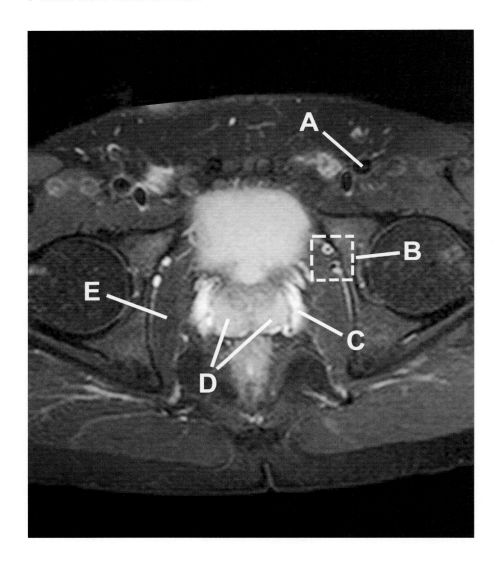

Q20

a Name the structure labelled A
b Name the structure labelled B
c Name the motor nerve supplying the structure labelled C
d Name the structure labelled D
e Name the structure labelled E

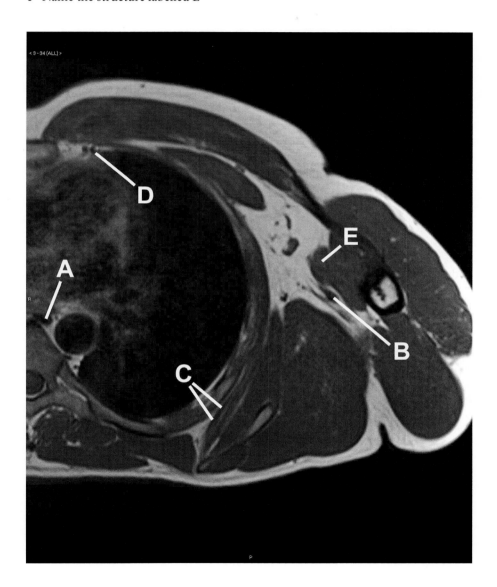

Q1 Answers

a Sacral nerve roots in sacral canal (cauda equina)
b Fat in the presacral space
c Rectal folds (valves)
d Posterior fornix of vagina
e Junctional zone of the myometrium

T2W MRI of female pelvis, midline sagittal section

The spinal cord terminates at the conus which is normally sited at the L1/2 level. The distal lumbar and sacral nerve roots leave the cord at the conus and collectively form the cauda equina (due to their somewhat similar appearance to a horse's tail) within the vertebral canal.

Physiological fluid and the mucosal surfaces of the uterus, cervix and vagina produce high signal on T2 which makes these collapsed cavities visible.

Q2 Answers

a Tendon of biceps brachii muscle
b Coronoid process of ulna
c Biceps brachii and brachialis
d Olecranon fossa
e Medial and lateral (ulnar and radial) collateral ligaments

Radiographs of elbow, AP and lateral views

The major flexors of the elbow are the biceps brachii and brachialis muscles which lie within the anterior humeral compartment. Their action is aided by the brachioradialis muscle (particularly when the forearm is in the mid-prone position), the belly of which is contained within the forearm.

The elbow joint is stabilized medially and laterally by strong collateral ligaments which originate from the epicondyles of the humerus. These are also known as the radial and ulnar collateral ligaments. The radial collateral ligament is continuous with the annular ligament of the radius. The ulnar collateral ligament has three discrete bands; anterior, posterior and oblique joining it to the coronoid process and olecranon of the ulna.

Q3 Answers

a Gastro-oesophageal junction
b Crus of right hemi-diaphragm
c Right colic flexure (hepatic flexure)
d Tail of the pancreas
e Left ureter

CT of upper abdomen with contrast, oblique coronal section

The two diaphragmatic crura arise from the upper lumbar vertebrae (L1/2/3 on the right and L1/2 on the left) and arch superiorly and anteriorly to form the margins of the aortic and oesophageal hiatuses. They are connected anteriorly by the median arcuate ligament which forms the anterior border of the aortic hiatus (T12). Anterior to this is the oesophageal hiatus (T10). The third and most anterior diaphragmatic hiatus is for the IVC (T8) which is situated immediately inferior to the right atrium within the large central tendon of the diaphragm.

Q4 Answers

a Left gastric artery
b Latissimus dorsi
c Aorto-pulmonary window
d Trachea
e Double SVC

CT thorax with contrast, maximum intensity projection, coronal section

In the developing venous system, paired superior cardinal veins drain into the two horns of the sinus venosus. The left horn develops into the coronary sinus and the right horn is incorporated into the right atrium. The upper cardinal veins interconnect via an oblique vein which becomes the left brachiocephalic vein. The inferior aspect of the left-sided cardinal vein usually involutes leaving a single, right-sided superior vena cava draining into the heart.

Failure to form an oblique vein results in a double SVC without communication. Involution of the right cardinal vein rather than the left results in a left SVC, and formation of an oblique vein but with no involution results in a double SVC with communication (as in this case). In most cases, a left SVC will drain into the coronary sinus.

Davies M, Guest PJ. Developmental abnormalities of the great vessels of the thorax and their embryological basis. *British Journal of Radiology* 2003; 76:491–502.

Q5 Answers

a Corpus callosum
b Right head of caudate
c Anterior limb left internal capsule
d Right internal carotid artery within cavernous sinus
e Septum pellucidum

T2W MRI of brain, coronal section at level of cavernous sinus

In coronal section the corpus callosum is clearly seen connecting the white matter of the two cerebral hemispheres. Similarly, the limbs of the internal capsule are seen to radiate from central to peripheral; the anterior limb lies anterior to the midline of the brains long axis which roughly corresponds with the position of the midbrain (the image provided is anterior to the brainstem).

The carotid artery turns through 180 degrees within the cavernous sinus before exiting superiorly and dividing into its terminal branches.

Q6 Answers

a Natal cleft
b Ischiopubic ramus
c Sartorius and tensor fascia latae
d Sacral ala (or wing)
e L5/S1 joint (or interspace)

Radiograph of male pelvis, AP view

Many soft tissue shadows are seen overlying the bony structures on plain radiography. These need to be recognised to exclude them from bony lucencies; soft tissue shadows will generally extend beyond the boundaries of the bone they overlie.

The pubis joins the ilium and ischium through superior (iliopubic) and inferior (ischiopubic) rami.

The sacral alae (or wings) are the lateral expansions of the sacrum which articulate with the ilium bilaterally.

Q7 Answers

a Medial tibial condyle
b Intercondylar fossa
c Base of the patella
d Adductor tubercle
e Soleus

Radiograph of knee, AP view

Parts of the patella are named in accordance with their shape, rather than the positions in which they are found in vivo. The base forms the flatter superior aspect and the apex lies inferiorly.

Soleus muscle is one of the three superficial calf muscles, and the only muscle to arise from both the proximal fibula and tibia. It takes origin from the upper fibula, including the head, as well as from the soleal line which is a thick oblique ridge on the posterior aspect of the upper tibia. The origins are connected by a fibrous band that passes over the popliteal vessels in the posterior calf. Soleus contains a large number of small perforating veins to the great saphenous vein. It plays an important role in maintaining venous flow by forcing blood from deep veins within the calf through these perforators to superficial veins every time the muscle belly contracts and therefore acts as a 'venous pump' in the lower limb.

Meissner MH, Moneta G, Burnand K *et al*. The hemodynamics and diagnosis of venous disease. *Journal of Vascular Surgery* 2007; 46: S4–S24.

Q8 Answers

a Right pedicle of T1 vertebra
b Coronoid process of mandible
c Inferior nasal concha (or turbinate)
d Ethmoid sinus
e Mastoid air cells

Radiograph of mandible, AP view

The midline part of the mandible is known as the body and has the mandibular protuberance anteriorly (the point of the chin). The mandibular rami are the more vertical lateral components of the mandible; the angle of the mandible is where the ramus meets the body, there are two of these. Both the condylar and coronoid processes of the mandible arise from the ramus. The condylar process articulates within the mandibular fossa of the temporal bone to form the temporomandibular joint (TMJ). The coronoid process arises more anteriorly and provides attachment for the temporalis, one of the four muscles of mastication.

Q9 Answers

a Aortic valve
b Lesser omentum
c Left brachiocephalic vein
d Spleen
e Left atrium/auricle

MRI of the aortic root, oblique coronal section

The lesser omentum consists of two layers of peritoneum which extends between the posterior aspect of the liver and the lesser curvature of the stomach. The hepatic connection is 'L'-shaped as it joins into the fissure for the ligamentum venosum and porta hepatis. The lesser omentum runs from the right side of the intrathoracic oesophagus, along the lesser curvature of the stomach and includes the first two centimetres of duodenum. The free edge at this point forms the anterior margin of the foramen of Winslow (epiploic foramen) and the lesser omentum is the anterior boundary of the lesser sac.

The thyroid is supplied by paired inferior thyroid arteries (from the thyrocervical trunk) and paired superior thyroid arteries (from the external carotid artery). In a small percentage of people there is a further artery supplying the thyroid – thyroidea ima – which arises directly either from the brachiocephalic trunk or the arch of the aorta.

Summers JE. Surgical anatomy of the thyroid gland. *Am Joint Surg* 1950; 80:35–43.

Q10 Answers

a Intermediate (middle) cuneiform
b Calcaneus
c Cuboid
d Epiphysis of 1st metatarsal
e Medial malleolus of the tibia

Radiographs of the foot in a 7 year-old child, AP and oblique views

The bones of the foot consist of the tarsus, metatarsus and phalanges. Tarsal bones of the foot are arranged in two rows. The proximal row consists of the calcaneus and talus. The distal row includes the medial, intermediate and lateral cuneiform bones medially and the cuboid laterally. On the medial side the navicular is positioned between the talus proximally and the cuneiforms distally.

Q11 Answers

a Vastus medialis
b Biceps femoris
c Sartorius
d Adductor canal (Hunter's canal, subsartorial canal)
e Linea aspera

T1W MRI of lower thigh, axial section

The adductor canal is a continuation from the apex of the femoral triangle. It is a channel that runs down the medial and lower thigh located between vastus medialis anteriorly, the adductors posteriorly and the sartorius medially. It serves to transmit the superficial femoral artery (and descending genicular branch) and femoral vein between the thigh and the popliteal fossa. To enter the popliteal fossa, the femoral artery turns medially and passes posteriorly through an opening in the aponeurosis of adductor magnus (adductor hiatus). The femoral vein lies deep to the artery throughout the thigh, but superficial to it in the popliteal fossa. The saphenous nerve enters the canal superiorly before exiting medially between sartorius and gracilis.

The linea aspera is a roughened ridge on the posterior aspect of the femoral shaft which receives the attachments of the biceps femoris (short head) and the abductor muscles.

Q12 Answers

a Trapezius muscle
b Anatomical neck of humerus
c Supraspinatus, infraspinatus, teres minor and subscapularis
d Lower border of teres major
e Axillary, radial, ulnar, median and musculocutaneous nerves

T1W MRI of shoulder, coronal section

The trapezius muscle (upper fibres) is used to shrug the shoulders by raising and rotating the scapula and raising the distal clavicle. It attaches distally to the lateral third of clavicle, acromion and spine of scapula.

The brachial vessels of the arm are continuous with the axillary vessels; they leave the axilla by passing distal to the lower border of teres major.

Most nerve supply to the upper limb derives from the brachial plexus. The nerve roots of C5 to T1 combine and cross before the five terminal nerves are formed. These nerves enter the arm surrounding the brachial artery.

Q13 Answers

a Left gonadal (testicular) vein
b Jejunum
c Iliacus
d Ileo-colic artery
e Left sub-phrenic space

CT abdomen with contrast, coronal section

In males, the testicular veins enter the abdominal cavity through the inguinal canal and run along the anterior aspect of the psoas muscle, usually in a pair either side of the testicular artery. The vein on the right empties into the IVC but on the left it usually inserts at a right angle into the left renal vein.

The superior mesenteric artery supplies the mid-gut structures, which includes bowel from half way along the 2nd part of duodenum to the distal two thirds of the transverse colon. Three branches of the SMA provide the colonic supply – the ileo-colic, right colic and middle colic arteries.

The left sub-phrenic space is separated from the right sub-phrenic space by the falciform ligament of the liver.

Q14 Answers

a Interosseous membrane
b Ulnar styloid
c Hook of hamate
d Epiphysis of thumb metacarpal
e Superficial and deep palmar arches

Radiograph of the wrist in a 13 year-old child, AP view

All carpal bones are visible in this image of an adolescent child and are almost fully ossified. The long bone epiphyses are similarly nearing their final size prior to fusion of the physes.

Q15 Answers

a Sternal and clavicular heads of sternocleidomastoid muscle
b Sternothryoid and sternohyoid muscles (strap muscles)
c Oesophagus
d Lamina
e Dorsal roots/ dorsal root ganglia of cervical cord

T2W MRI at root of neck, axial section

The sternocleidomastoid (SCM) muscle has, as the name suggests, a sternal and clavicular head. Medial to the SCM lie the strap muscles. These are named by their attachments; the sternothyroid lies deep to the sternohyoid. The strap muscles depress the hyoid and larynx.

Each spinal nerve is formed from dorsal and ventral nerve roots which combine as they leave the vertebral canal. The dorsal nerve root is sensory and its nerve cell bodies are contained within the dorsal root ganglion. The ventral nerve roots are motor and have their ganglia within the spinal cord. After leaving the vertebral canal, a spinal nerve almost immediately divides into dorsal and ventral rami which supply the posterior and anterior parts of the body, respectively.

Q16 Answers

a Anterior leaflet (cusp) of the mitral valve
b Papillary muscle
c Left breast
d Left coronary artery
e Left atrium

Cardiac MRI (Gradient Echo/True fast imaging with steady state precession (True FISP)), long-axis vertical plane

This long axis vertical plane view demonstrates the left atrium and ventricle. Horizontal long axis (or 4-chamber view) and short-axis plane can also be used specifically for cardiac MRI.

The orientation of the heart means that there is significant obliquity in the projection of the extra-cardiac structures. The lower part of the image is significantly further left than the upper part.

This image is taken in early systole, shortly after closure of the mitral valve.

Lee VS. Cardiac MRI: Technical Aspects and Primer. *Radiology* 2002; eMedicine: www.emedicine.medscape.com

Q17 Answers

a Interosseous sacroiliac ligament
b Dorsal nerve root
c Nerve roots of the cauda equina
d Dorsal sacroiliac ligament
e Gluteus medius

T2W MRI of lower lumbar spine, axial section

Each sacro-iliac joint has to withstand significant forces as they support the axial load of the trunk through their connection to the pelvis and lower limb. The adjacent joint surfaces are irregular but reciprocal in outline which adds to this strength. Additional support is provided by dorsal and ventral sacroiliac ligaments and a deeper interosseous sacroiliac ligament. A small amount of movement is permitted in the joint, predominantly in a rotatory axis.

Nerve roots exit the dura mater to pass obliquely and inferiorly through the intervertebral foramina.

Q18 Answers

a Anterior lobe of the cerebellum
b Clivus
c Uvula
d Posterior arch of C1
e C4/5 level

T2W MRI of neck, midline sagittal section

On this view the anterior lobe of the cerebellum is visible divided from the posterior lobe by the CSF filled primary fissure. The third major lobe of the cerebellum is the flocculonodular lobe which lies antero-inferiorly.

There are thirty-one pairs of spinal nerves. These exit the spinal canal through the intervertebral foramen which are formed from notches in the superior and inferior pedicles of adjacent vertebrae. The individual nerves are named relative to these adjacent vertebrae; cervical nerves are named relative to the inferior pedicle of their foramen, however since there are eight cervical nerves but only seven cervical vertebrae, the eighth cervical spinal nerve exits below the seventh cervical vertebra. The remaining spinal nerves (thoracic, lumbar and sacral) are named relative to the superior pedicle of their foramen, i.e. T7 exits at the T7/8 level.

Q19 Answers

a Common femoral artery
b Obturator artery, vein and nerve
c Seminal vesicle
d Peripheral zone of prostate
e Obturator internus muscle

T2W MRI of male pelvis with fat saturation, axial section

On this image, the urinary bladder is seen in the midline with the prostate beneath. Prostatic zonal anatomy is well seen with the higher signal peripheral zone surrounding the lower signal central gland. Superior and lateral to the prostate on either side of the midline lie the seminal vesicles.

The iliac vessels are continuous distally with the common femoral vessels; the name changes as they pass under the inguinal ligament and leave the pelvis. The obturator vessels are branches of the anterior division of the internal iliac vessels. The obturator vessels run along the lateral wall of the pelvis. Initially they lie medial to the obturator internus muscle but distally they perforate this layer to reach the obturator foramen.

Q20 Answers

a Azygous vein
b Axillary artery/brachial artery
c Long thoracic nerve
d Internal mammary artery
e Teres major

T1W MRI of the thorax at the level of the left axilla, axial section

The axillary artery passes through the axilla alongside the axillary vein, which lies medial to the cords of the brachial plexus; these surround the artery and are named according to their position relative to it.

As the axillary artery crosses the inferior border of teres major it is renamed the brachial artery.

The long thoracic nerve is a branch of the upper roots of the brachial plexus, arising from the posterior aspects of C5/6/7. It travels inferiorly along the superficial fascia of serratus anterior. The action of serratus anterior is that of a powerful lateral rotator (lower half) and protractor of the scapula.

The internal mammary artery, which is a branch of the subclavian artery, passes down behind the first six costal cartilages on the inner anterior thoracic wall. The artery is located lateral to the vein.

INDEX

Note: page numbers in parentheses refer to questions. Other page numbers refer to answers.

abdominal wall muscles (162) 178
abductor digiti mimimi muscle 244
abductor hallucis muscle (229) 244
aberrant pulmonary arteries 103
aberrant right subclavian artery (88) 111
abscesses, ischioanal 208
accessory fissures (pleura) 96
accessory hemiazygos vein 109
accessory nerve, spinal (90) 112
acetabular angle (213) 233
acetabulum (183) 202, (212) 232
    child (215) 234–5
    triradiate cartilage (213) 233
Achilles tendon (226) 242, (231) 245
acromio-clavicular joint (117) 137, (119) 138
acromion process, scapula (116) 136, (121) 139
acute marginal branch artery (76) 102
Adam's apple 55
adductor brevis muscle 237
adductor canal (256) 271
adductor hiatus 271
adductor longus muscle 237
adductor magnus muscle 237, (218) 237
adductor tubercle (252) 269
adolescents, carpal bones (259) 272
adrenal gland (156) 174, (164) 179
age
    gestational 206
    physiological 145
alpha angle, paediatric hip (215) 234, 235
ambient cistern (12) 47
ampulla of Vater (151) 171, 181
ampulla, fallopian tube 204
anastomoses
    axillary artery (122) 139
    brain arteries 49
    lower limb arteries 234
    porto-systemic 176
anatomical neck, humerus 136, (257) 271
angle of Louis 101
angle of mandible (26) 55
ankle joint (226 & 227) 242–3, (229) 244
annular ligament (125) 141
annulus fibrosus 113–14
anterior cerebral artery (12) 47
anterior clinoid process (5) 43

anterior descending coronary artery (82) 107, (84) 108
anterior fontanelle (5) 43
anterior humeral line (126) 141
anterior inferior iliac spine (183) 202, 232
anterior inferior talofibular ligament (228) 243
anterior meniscofemoral ligament (223) 240
anterior sacral foramina (184) 202
anterior superior iliac spine 232
anterior temporal lobe (25) 54
anterior tibial artery (221) 239
anterior vertebral line (29) 57
antrum, stomach (151) 170, 174
anus, external sphincter (194) 207
aorta
    abdominal (149) 169, (160) 176, (192) 206, (201) 211
    arch (39) 62, (65) 95, (77) 103, (81) 106
    descending (71) 99
    root (254) 270
aortic hiatus 267
aortic valve (69) 98, (83) 108, (254) 270
aorto-pulmonary window (249) 267
aponeuroses
    bicipital 141
    external oblique muscle (162) 178
    palmar (135) 146
    plantar (230) 244
appendix (153) 172
aqueduct of Sylvius (20) 51, (22) 53
arachnoid layer, meninges 49
arcuate ligament 241
    median 267
arcuate line 178
areola (74) 101
arteries
    brain 49
    end-on (lung) 96
    see also named arteries
arteries of Riolan 173
artery of Adamkiewicz (167) 181, 182
arthrography, wrist 144
arytenoid cartilages 59
ascending colon (153) 172
atlanto-axial joint (28) 56
atlas (C1) (6) 44, (27 & 28) 56, (31 & 32) 58
    posterior arch (263) 274
atria (64) 94, (80) 106, (82) 107, (83) 108, (254) 270, (261) 273
atrio-ventricular node 107

avascular necrosis, femoral head 234
axillary artery (81) 106, 107, (93) 115, (120) 138, (122) 139, (265) 275
axillary lymph nodes (75) 102, 115
axillary nerve (120) 138, 139, (257) 271
axillary vein (118) 137, (120) 138, 275
axis (C2) (28) 56, (29) 57, 58
azygo-oesophageal line (69) 98
azygos fissure (67) 96
azygos lobe 96
azygos vein (85) 109, (265) 275

barium small-bowel follow-through (151) 170–1
barium swallow (77) 103, (78) 104
basal ganglia (19) 51
basilar artery (16) 49, (17) 50
basilic vein 140, 143
basivertebral veins (167) 181, 182
beta angle, paediatric hip (215) 234, 235
biceps brachii muscle (120) 138, (123) 140, (247) 266
    long head tendon (116) 136, (118) 137
biceps femoris muscle 237, (256) 271
    tendon (224) 240–1
bicipital aponeurosis 141
Bigelow's ligament (212) 232
biliary system (166) 180–1
bipartite patella 238
bladder (188) 204, (190) 205, (196) 208, (200) 210
Bohler's angle (226) 242
bone marrow (87) 110–11
bovine arch (81) 106
brachial artery (122) 139, (128) 142, (265) 275
brachial plexus (39) 62, (92) 114, (257) 271
brachial vein (124) 140
brachialis muscle (123) 140, (247) 266
brachiocephalic artery 100
brachiocephalic vein, left 267, (254) 270
brachioradialis muscle 266
brain (12) 47, (16) 49, (250) 268
    neonate (14) 48, (15) 49
    vascular system 49
breast (65) 95, (74) 101, (75) 102, (261) 273
    carcinoma, axillary lymph nodes 115
bregma 43
broad ligament (192) 206
bronchi (77) 103, (85) 109, (86) 110
    end-on 96
bronchopulmonary segments 104–5, 109
bronchus intermedius (67) 96, 110
bulbospongiosus muscle (194) 207, 208
bulbous urethra 204, (188) 204

caecum 172
calcaneum 245, (255) 270
    fractures 242
calyces, kidney (161) 177, (185) 203
capitate (132) 144, (133) 145
capitulum, humerus (125) 141, (127) 142
capsule, knee joint (223) 240
cardia, stomach 174
cardiac fat pad (72) 100
cardinal veins, superior 267

cardiophrenic angles (65) 95
carina 95
carotid arteries (81) 106, (250) 268
    common carotid artery 62
    external carotid artery (36) 60, (40) 62, 63
    internal carotid artery 59, (36) 60, 62–3, (250) 268
carotid canal (9) 45
carpal bones 143, 144, (133) 145, (259) 272
carpal tunnel 145
cauda equina 205, (246) 266, (262) 274
caudate lobe, liver (164) 179
caudate nucleus (12) 47, (250) 268
caval opening, diaphragm (80) 106
cavernous sinuses 47, (250) 268
cavum septum pellucidum (14) 48, 50
cephalic vein (123) 140, (124) 140, (129) 143
cerebellar peduncles (13) 48, (21) 52, (25) 54–5, (90) 112
cerebello-pontine angle (24) 54
cerebellum (21) 52, (263) 274
cerebral aqueduct (20) 51, (22) 53
cerebral hemispheres (15) 49
cerebral peduncles 49
cerebrospinal fluid 47
cervical rib 55, (68) 97
cervical spine (1) 41, (26) 55, (27 & 28) 56, (29) 57, (31) 58
cervix uteri (187) 204, (190) 205, (197) 209
chest wall muscles (88) 111
children
    carpal bones (259) 272
    elbow (127) 142
    hip joint (215) 234–5
    knee joint (220) 238
    paranasal sinuses (1) 41
    pelvis (213) 233
    physiological age 145
    skull (5) 43
choanae 58
chorion (191) 206
cingulate gyrus (14) 48
circle of Willis 49
circumflex coronary artery 107
circumflex humeral vessels 139, (122) 139
cisterns (brain)
    ambient cistern (12) 47
    pontine cistern (13) 48
claustrum (19) 51
clavicle (73) 100, (92) 114, (117) 137, (120) 138
clinoid processes (5) 43
clivus (9) 45, (263) 274
coccygeus muscle (198) 209
coccyx (183) 202
cochlea (24) 54
cochlear nerve (24) 54
coeliac artery 171, (154) 172
collateral arteries, arm 139
collateral ligaments
    elbow joint (247) 266–7
    knee joint (224) 240
collecting system, renal (161) 177
colliculi (superior & inferior) 49, (20) 51, (20 & 21) 52

colon (153) 172, (159) 176
  blood supply 173
  descending (147) 168
  haustra (148) 168
  hepatic flexure (248) 267
columns see three column principle
columns of Bertin (165) 180
common bile duct (163) 178, (164) 179, (166) 180
common carotid artery 62
common femoral artery (214) 234, (264) 275
common femoral vein (216) 235
common hepatic artery (152) 171
common iliac artery (149) 169, 177, (185) 203, (201) 211
common iliac vein (185) 203
common peroneal nerve 236
compartments, leg (225) 241, 242, 243
conchae (inferior nasal) (23) 53, (253) 269
condylar process, mandible (6) 44, (8) 45, (254) 269
condyles, tibia (252) 269
confluence of sinuses (11) 46–7
conoid component, coracoclavicular ligament (116) 136
conus branch, coronary arteries (76) 102
conus medullaris (167) 181
Cooper's ligaments (74) 101
coracoclavicular ligament (116) 136
coracoid process, scapula (70) 99, (117) 137, (120) 138
corniculate cartilages 59
coronal sections, shoulder (120) 138
coronal suture (5) 43
coronary arteries (76) 102–3, (82) 107, (83) 108, (261)
    273
  anterior descending coronary artery (82) 107, (84)
    108
  posterior descending coronary artery (76) 102, 103,
    (81) 106, 107
coronoid process
  mandible (3) 42, (253) 269
  ulna (126) 141, (247) 266
corpora cavernosa 207
corpora quadrigemina 49, (20) 51, (22) 52, (20 & 21) 52
corpus callosum (17 & 18) 50, (250) 268
corpus spongiosum 207
cortex, skull 43
costophrenic recess (72) 100
costotransverse joints 110
costovertebral joints (87) 110
Couinaud, C., hepatic segments 173
cranial fossae 46
cranial nerves, in cavernous sinuses 47
cribriform plates 46
cricoid cartilage 59
cricothyroid ligament 55
cricothyroid membrane 55, (33) 59
CRITOE (mnemonic) 142
crown rump length (191) 206
crowns, teeth (7) 44
cruciate ligaments, posterior (223) 240, (224) 240
crus cerebri (22) 52
cuboid (226) 242, (255) 270
cuneiform bones (231) 245, (255) 270
cuneiform cartilages 59
cystic duct 180

d/D ratio, paediatric hip 235
deep brachial artery (122) 139, (123) 140
deep brachial vein (123) 140, (124) 140
deep circumflex iliac artery (201) 211
deep palmar arch (128) 142, (259) 272
deltoid ligament 243, (229) 244
deltoid muscle (118) 137, (119) 138
dens 55, (27 & 28) 56, (31) 58
dentine (7) 44
dermatomes, foot (231) 245
descending aorta (71) 99
descending colon (147) 168
developmental dysplasia of hip 233, 235
diaphragm (64 & 65) 94, 95, (69) 98, (71) 99, (156) 174,
    (165) 180, (248) 267
  caval opening (80) 106
diaphragma sellae 43
diaphyses, femur (220) 238
digital arteries, palmar (135) 146
discs (intervertebral) (91) 113–14
distal radioulnar joint (130) 143
distal tibiofibular joint 243
dorsal pancreatic duct (166) 180, 181
dorsal root ganglia (91) 113
dorsal sacroiliac ligament (262) 274
dorsal scapular artery (90) 112
dorsal spinal nerve roots
  cervical (260) 273
  lumbar (262) 274
dorsum sellae (10) 46
double inferior vena cava (160) 176–7
double superior vena cava (249) 267
duct of Santorini (166) 180, 181
duct of Wirsung 181
ductus venosus (149) 169
duodenocolic ligament (157) 174
duodenum (151) 170–1, (154) 172, (157) 174
duplication, inferior vena cava (160) 176–7
dura mater 49
dysphagia lusoria 111

edges, lines vs, pleural reflections 98
ejaculatory ducts 204
elbow (125 & 126) 141, (127) 142
elbow joint (247) 266
  collateral ligaments (247) 266–7
enamel (7) 44
endocervical canal (197) 209
endometrium (190) 205, (197) 209
epicardial fat (84) 108, 109
epicondyles
  femur (219) 238
  humerus 141, (127) 142
epididymis (193) 206, 207
epidural fat (167) 181
epiglottis (33) 59, (35) 60, (37) 61
epiphyseal lines (119) 138
epiphyses
  elbow (127) 142
  femur (220) 238
  fingers (134) 145

first metacarpal (259) 272
  tibia (220) 238
epiploic foramen (158) 175
erectile tissue, penis (194) 207
erector spinae muscles (87) 110
ethmoid sinuses (253) 269
  posterior (23) 53
extensor digitorum muscle (228) 243
extensor hallucis longus muscle 243, (230) 244
extensor paraspinal muscles 110
extensors, leg (225) 241
external capsule (19) 51
external carotid artery (36) 60, (40) 62, 63
external iliac artery (161) 177, (195) 208
external oblique muscle 178
  aponeurosis (162) 178
external sphincter, anus (194) 207
extra-ocular muscles (23) 53
extreme capsule (19) 51
eye muscles (extra-ocular muscles) (23) 53

fabella (222) 239
facet joints (zygoapophyseal joints) (27) 56, (91) 113, (150) 169
facial bones, occipito-mental view (3) 42
facial nerve (24) 54, (36) 60-1
falciform ligament, liver 272
fallopian tube (187) 204
falx cerebri (14) 48, (15) 49
fascia lata 237
fascia of Zuckerkandl (160) 176, 177
fat pads
  cardiac (72) 100
  elbow (126) 141
  infrapatellar (222) 239
female pelvis 202, (185) 203, (196) 208
female reproductive tract, ultrasound (190) 205, (191) 206
femoral artery (216) 235, 271
femoral canal (216) 235
femoral head (215) 234, (216) 235
femoral nerve 236
femoral vein 235, 236, 271
femur
  epicondyles (219) 238
  greater trochanter (217) 236
  linea aspera (256) 271
  ossification 235, (220) 238
fillings, dental (7) 44, (28) 56
fistula, perianal 208
flexor digitorum brevis 244
flexor digitorum longus 242-3
flexor digitorum profundus, tendons (133) 145, 146
flexor digitorum superficialis, tendons (133) 145, (135) 146
flexor hallucis longus muscle (227) 242-3, (230) 244
flexor pollicis longus (133) 145
flexor retinaculum (133) 145
flexors, forearm (125) 141, (129) 143, 146
flocculonodular lobe, cerebellum 274
foetal circulation 169
foetus (191) 206
folia, cerebellum (21) 52

follicles, ovary (192) 206
fontanelles (5) 43
foot
  dermatomes (231) 245
  tarsal bones (231) 245, (255) 270
foramen lacerum (40) 62
foramen magnum (4) 42-3, (9) 45, (35) 60
foramen of Monro (19) 51
foramen of Winslow (158) 175
foramen ovale (8) 45
foramen rotundum (2) 42, (8) 45
foramen spinosum (8) 45
fornices (white matter) (18) 50
fornices, vagina 209, (246) 266
fourth ventricle (13) 48, 52
  superior medullary velum (35) 60
frontal bone (10) 46
frontal process, zygoma (8) 45
frontal sinus (1) 41, (2) 42, (18) 51
fronto-zygomatic suture (3) 42
fundus, stomach (71) 99, (78) 104, 174

gallbladder (155) 173, (163) 178, (166) 180
  non-opacification 181
ganglia, dorsal spinal nerve roots (91) 113, (260) 273
gastro-oesophageal junction (78) 104, (248) 267
gastrocnemius muscle (222) 239, (225) 241, 245
gastroduodenal artery (152) 171
gastrosplenic ligament (158) 175
genu of corpus callosum (18) 50
genu of internal capsule (12) 47
Gerota's fascia 177
gestational age 206
gestational sac (191) 206
gleno-humeral joint (119) 138
glenoid cavity (117) 137
glenoid labrum (119) 138
globus pallidus (19) 51
gluteus medius muscle (262) 274
golfer's elbow 141
gonadal artery (161) 177, 206, (201) 211
  see also ovarian artery; testicular artery
gonadal vein (258) 272
gracilis muscle 237
great longitudinal fissure (14) 48
great saphenous vein (216) 235, (224) 240, 241, (227) 242
greater trochanter (217) 236

hamate (133) 145, (259) 272
hamstrings, origin (218) 237
hand
  blood supply (128) 142
  bone development (134) 145
hard palate 51
haustra, colon (148) 168
heart (64) 94, (84) 108-9
  MRI (261) 273
  valves see valves (cardiac)
  see also coronary arteries; ventricles
hemiazygos vein 109
hepatic artery (163) 178, 179

hepatic bile ducts (166) 180
hepatic flexure of colon (248) 267
hepatic segments (155) 173
hepatic veins (163) 178, 179
hepato-renal pouch (160) 176, 177
hepatoduodenal ligament 175
hilar point (69) 98
Hilgenreiner line (213) 233
hip joint 232, (213) 233
    blood supply 234
    child (215) 234–5
    ligamentum teres (195) 208
hippocampus (17) 50
Hoffa's fat pad (222) 239
hook of hamate (259) 272
horizontal fissure (pleura) (67) 96
Houston, valves of (186) 203
humerus (116) 136
    anatomical neck 136, (257) 271
    capitulum (125) 141, (127) 142
    epicondyles 141, (127) 142
    medulla (123) 140
    olecranon fossa (126) 141, (247) 266
Humphrey's ligament (223) 240
Hunter's canal (256) 271
hydrocele (193) 207
hyoid bone (26) 55, (30) 57, (33) 59
hypoglossal nerve (9) 45, (37) 61
hypothenar eminence (133) 145
hysterosalpingography (187) 204

ileocolic artery 173, (258) 272
ileum (151) 170
    blood supply 173
iliacus muscle (195) 208, (258) 272
iliofemoral ligament (212) 232
iliopsoas muscles (189) 205, (217) 236
iliotibial tract 237, 240–1
incisors (6) 44
incisura (cardiac) (72) 100
incisura (stomach) (156) 174
inferior alveolar artery and nerve 44
inferior colliculi 49, (20) 51, (20 & 21) 52
inferior epigastric artery (201) 211
inferior gluteal artery 234
inferior mesenteric artery 171, (154) 172–3, (201) 211
inferior nasal concha (23) 53, (253) 269
inferior petrosal sinus 47
inferior rectal artery (186) 203
inferior rectus muscle (23) 53
inferior sagittal sinus (11) 46–7
inferior vena cava (71) 99, (149) 169, (164) 179
    diaphragmatic hiatus 267
    double (160) 176–7
infra-mammary skin fold (75) 102
infrapatellar fat pad (222) 239
infraspinatus muscle (88) 111, (118) 137, (257) 271
infundibulum, fallopian tube 204
inguinal canal 236
innominate bone 202, 233
innominate line (2) 42
insula (14) 48, (17) 50

interatrial septum (82) 107
intercondylar eminence, tubercle of (219) 238
intercondylar fossa (252) 269
intercostal arteries 182
intercostal muscles (88) 111
interhemispheric fissure (14) 48
interlobar arteries (80) 106
intermediate cuneiform (231) 245
internal auditory meatus (24) 54
internal capsule (12) 47, 51, (250) 268
internal carotid artery 59, (36) 60, 62–3, (250) 268
internal cerebral veins (11) 46–7
internal iliac artery (149) 169, (192) 206, (201) 211
internal iliac vein (192) 206
internal jugular vein 59, (34) 59
internal mammary artery (81) 106, 107, (84) 108, (265) 275
internal oblique muscle (162) 178
internal pudendal artery 203
interosseous arteries, forearm (128) 142
interosseous ligament 243
interosseous membrane
    forearm (129) 143, (259) 272
    leg (225) 241
interosseous sacroiliac ligament (262) 274
interosseous talocalcaneal ligament (229) 244
interosseous muscles
    foot (230) 244
    hand 146
interpeduncular cistern (13) 48, (22) 52
interspinous ligaments (1) 41
intertubercular groove (118) 137
interventricular septum (89) 112
intervertebral discs (91) 113–14
intervertebral foramina 114, (150) 169
intra-conal fat (16) 49
intra-uterine contraceptive devices (185) 203
ischial spine (184) 202
ischioanal fossa 208, (218) 237
ischiocavernosus muscle (194) 207, 208
ischiopubic ramus (251) 268
ischiopubic synchondrosis (213) 233
isthmus of fallopian tube 204
isthmus of thyroid gland (34) 59

jejunal branch, superior mesenteric artery (155) 173
jejunum (151) 170, 171, (258) 272
Judet views 232
jugular foramen (9) 45

kidney (147) 168, (161) 177, (165) 180, (185) 203
    renal pelvis (152) 171, 177
knee joint (219) 238, (222) 239, (223 & 224) 240–1, (252) 269
    child (220) 238

labrum (of glenoid) (119) 138
lambda 43
lambdoid suture (5) 43, (10) 46
lamina dura (7) 44
lamina papyracea (3) 42
laminae, vertebrae (87) 110, 170, (260) 273

large intestine (153) 172
laryngopharynx (32) 58
larynx (33) 59
   cartilages (26) 55, (27) 56
lateral circumflex femoral artery (214) 234
lateral mass of atlas (31) 58
lateral meniscus (223) 240
lateral pterygoid muscle (36) 60
lateral sulcus (sylvian fissure) (13 & 14) 48, (17) 50
lateral ventricles, temporal horns (16) 49
latissimus dorsi muscle (249) 267
left atrium (254) 270
   appendage (80) 106, (82) 107
left brachiocephalic vein 267, (254) 270
left colic artery 173
left gastric artery (78) 104, (249) 267
left hepatic artery (152) 171
lentiform nucleus (19) 51
lesser omentum (254) 270
lesser sac (158) 175
lesser tubercle, humerus (116) 136
lesser wing of sphenoid bone (10) 46
levator ani muscle (196) 208, (199) 210
lienorenal ligament (158) 175
ligament(s), thoracic spine 113
ligament of Bigelow (212) 232
ligament of Humphrey (223) 240
ligament of ovary (192) 206
ligament of Treitz 171
ligamentum arteriosum (79) 104, 105
ligamentum flavum (1) 41, 113
ligamentum nuchae (91) 113
ligamentum teres, hip (195) 208
limbic system 50
linea alba (162) 178
linea aspera (256) 271
lines, edges vs, pleural reflections 98
lingula, bronchi supplying (85) 109
liver (147) 168, (158) 175, 178–9
   caudate lobe (164) 179
   neonatal (149) 169
   segments (155) 173
lobes (lung) (67) 96
long saphenous vein (216) 235, (224) 240, 241, (227)
   242
long thoracic nerve (265) 275
longitudinal ligaments (167) 181, 182
   cervical spine (1) 41
   thoracic spine 113
lumbar spine (150) 169–70, (262) 274
   lumbo-sacral junction (148) 169, 170
   transverse processes (148) 168
lumbarization, S1 vertebra (148) 169
lumbo-sacral joint (186) 203, (251) 268
lumbrical muscles (135) 146
lunate (130) 143, (132) 144
lung (67) 96
   bronchopulmonary segments 104–5, 109
   oblique fissure (72) 100, (85) 109
   right middle lobe (89) 112
lymph nodes
   axillary (75) 102, 115

breast 101
   mediastinum (68) 97, (77) 103

Magendie, median aperture of (20) 51
magnetic resonance imaging
   bone marrow 111
   gleno-humeral joint (119) 138
   heart (261) 273
   intervertebral discs 114
   orbit (16) 49
   pelvis (246) 266
   sacroiliac joint (199) 210
   shoulder (120) 138
   uterus (197) 209
male pelvis 202, (251) 268, (264) 275
malleoli (227) 242, (255) 270
mamillary body (20) 51–2
mammography (74) 101, (75) 102
mandible (253) 269
   angle (26) 55
   condylar process (6) 44, (8) 45, (254) 269
   coronoid process (3) 42, (253) 269
   orthopantomograms (6) 44
mandibular canal (6) 44
manubriosternal joint (73) 100, 101
manubrium (73) 100, 101, (92) 114
marrow (87) 110–11
massa intermedia, thalamus (20) 51
masseter muscle (36) 60
mastoid air cells (1) 41, (10) 46, (253) 269
maxillary ostium see inferior nasal concha
maxillary sinus (1) 41, (3) 42, (23) 53
McRae's line (35) 60
meati, nose (23) 53
Meckel's cave (25) 54–5
medial genicular artery (221) 239
medial intermuscular septum, thigh 237
medial pterygoid muscle (36) 60
medial tibial plateau (219) 238
medial tibial spine (219) 238
median aperture of Magendie (20) 51
median arcuate ligament 267
median nerve (133) 145, (257) 271
median sacral crest (189) 205
mediastinum (64 & 65) 94
   lymph nodes (68) 97, (77) 103
   pleural reflections (69) 98
mediastinum testis (193) 206
medulla, humerus (123) 140
membranous urethra (188) 204
meninges 49
menisci (knee) (223) 240
meniscofemoral ligament, anterior (223) 240
mesentery 172
mesorectal fascia (198) 209
metacarpals (134) 145, (259) 272
metaphyses (125) 141
   tibia (220) 238
metatarsals (255) 270
midbrain (16) 49
middle colic artery 173
middle ear (24) 54

middle meningeal artery
  foramen spinosum and (8) 45
  pterion and 43
middle rectal artery (186) 203
minor fissure (pleura) (67) 96
minor papilla 181
mitral valve (69) 98, (89) 112, (261) 273
moderator band, right ventricle (89) 112
Morison's pouch (160) 176, 177
musculocutaneous nerve (257) 271
mylohyoid muscle (32) 58
myometrium (190) 205, (191) 206, (246) 266
  junctional zone (197) 209

nasolacrimal duct 53
nasopharynx (32) 58
natal cleft (198) 209, (251) 268
navicular (231) 245, 270
neonate
  abdomen (149) 169
  brain (14) 48, (15) 49
  chest (70) 99
nerve roots see spinal nerve roots
neural arch of atlas (31) 58
neural foramina (intervertebral foramina) 114, (150) 169
nipple (75) 102
non-coronary sinus (82) 107
nose (23) 53
  inferior concha (23) 53, (253) 269
nucleus pulposus 113–14

oblique fissure (lung) (72) 100, (85) 109
oblique muscles, eye (23) 53
obturator artery (264) 275
obturator externus muscle (194) 207
obturator foramen (183) 202, 236
obturator internus muscle (195) 208, (199) 210, (264) 275
obturator nerve (217) 236, (264) 275
obturator vein (264) 275
occipito-frontal view, structures shown (2) 42
occipito-mental view, structures shown (3) 42
odontoid process (dens) 55, (27 & 28) 56, (31) 58
oesophageal hiatus 267
oesophagus (32) 58, (77) 103, (78) 104, (91) 113, (260) 273
olecranon fossa, humerus (126) 141, (247) 266
olecranon process, ulna (126) 141, 142
orbit (23) 53
  magnetic resonance imaging (16) 49
  occipito-mental view (3) 42
oropharynx 58, (37) 61
orthopantomograms (6) 44
ossification
  ASIS and AIIS 232
  coracoid process of scapula (70) 99
  femur (220) 238
    head 235
  forearm (127) 142
  hand (134) 145
  patella (220) 238
ostiomeatal complex (23) 53
ovarian artery (201) 211
  see also gonadal artery

ovarian ligament (192) 206
ovary (192) 206

palate 51
  see also soft palate
palmar aponeurosis (135) 146
palmar arches (128) 142, (259) 272
palmar digital arteries (135) 146
pancreas (157) 174, (164) 179, (248) 267
pancreas divisum (166) 180, 181
pancreatic duct 181
papilla of Vater (ampulla of Vater) (151) 171, 181
papillary muscles (83) 108, (261) 273
parahippocampal gyrus (17) 50
paranasal sinuses (1) 41, 51, (23) 53
parapharyngeal space (36) 60
pararectal fat (198) 209
paratracheal lymph nodes (68) 97
paratracheal stripe (65) 95
parotid gland (36) 60–1
pars interarticularis (150) 169, 170
patella (219) 238, (252) 269
  ossification (220) 238
pectineal line (183) 202
pectoralis major muscle (75) 102, (92) 114, (93) 115, 138
pectoralis minor muscle (88) 111, (93) 115
pedicles, vertebrae (87) 110, (253) 269
  cervical (30) 57
  lumbar (148) 168, 170
  thoracic (70) 99
peduncles, cerebellar (13) 48, (21) 52, (25) 54–5, (90) 112
pelvi-ureteric junction (161) 177, (185) 203
pelvic diaphragm 208, 209
pelvic floor (urogenital diaphragm) 204, (196) 208
pelvicalyceal system (161) 177
pelvis
  bony (183) 202, (212) 232, 233
  child (213) 233
  female 202, (185) 203, (196) 208
  male 202, (251) 268, (264) 275
  MRI (246) 266
penile urethra (188) 204
penis (184) 202, (194) 207
perianal fistula 208
pericardium 109
periodontal membranes (7) 44
perirectal fascia (198) 209
perirectal fat (198) 209
perirenal fat 177
peritoneum 174, 175
Perkins line 233
peroneal retinaculum (228) 243
peroneus brevis muscle 243
peroneus longus muscle (225) 241, (227) 242, 243, (229) 244, 245
peroneus tertius muscle 243
petrosal sinuses 47
petrous ridge (2) 42, (4) 43, 46
phalanges, fingers (134) 145
phrenic nerve (66) 95, (80) 106, (86) 110
phrenicocolic ligament (157) 174
physes, fingers (134) 145

pia mater 49
pisiform (131) 144, (133) 145
pituitary fossa (35) 60
plantar aponeurosis (230) 244
plantaris muscle 245
pleura (67) 96, (85) 109
pleural reflections, mediastinum (69) 98
pneumatization, paranasal sinuses (1) 41
pons (13) 48, (25) 54–5, (35) 60
pontine cistern (13) 48
popliteal artery (221) 238, 239
popliteal trifurcation 239
popliteus muscle (222) 239
popliteus tendon (219) 238, (222) 239
porta hepatis 179
portal triads 180
portal vein (149) 169, (159) 176, (163) 178, 179
porto-systemic anastomoses 176
posterior communicating arteries (16) 49
posterior descending coronary artery (76) 102, 103, (81) 106, 107
posterior fontanelle 43
posterior longitudinal ligament, cervical spine (1) 41
posterior renal fascia (160) 176, 177
posterior tibial artery (221) 238, 239, (225) 241
pouch of Douglas (197) 209
pregnancy, ultrasound (191) 206
presacral space (186) 203, (246) 266
presacral vertebra (148) 168
prevertebral soft tissues (27) 56
profunda brachii (deep brachial artery) (122) 139, (123) 140
profunda femoris artery (214) 234
prostate (195) 208, 210, (200) 210, (264) 275
prostatic urethra (188) 204, (200) 210
psoas major muscle (147) 168, 169, (160) 176, (165) 180
pterion (5) 43
pubic symphysis (184) 202, (213) 233
pubic tubercle (186) 203
pulmonary arteries (64) 94, (69) 98, 105, (84) 108, (86) 110
    aberrant 103
    interlobar (80) 106
    segmental (67) 96
pulmonary veins (69) 98, (79) 104, 105, (84) 108, (86) 110
pulp cavities, teeth (7) 44
putamen (19) 51
pyloric antrum, stomach (151) 170, 174
pyramids, renal (165) 180

quadrangular space 139
quadriceps femoris muscle 237

radial artery (128) 142, (129) 143
radial collateral ligament (247) 266–7
radial head (127) 142
radial nerve (123) 140, (129) 143, (257) 271
radial tuberosity (125) 141
radial vein (124) 140, (129) 143
radiculomedullary arteries 182
radius, styloid process (130) 143
recto-uterine pouch (197) 209

rectum (153) 172, (186) 203, (199) 210, (246) 266
rectus abdominis muscle (162) 178, (196) 208
rectus femoris muscle (183) 202, (212) 232, 237
rectus muscles, eye (23) 53
rectus sheath 178
recurrent laryngeal nerve (80) 106, (90) 112
red nucleus (22) 52, 53
renal artery (161) 177
renal pelvis (152) 171, 177
renal sinus (165) 180
renal veins (154) 172, (157) 174
rete testis (193) 206, 207
retro-areolar ducts (74) 101, (75) 102
retromandibular veins (36) 60, 61
retroperitoneal space 177
ribs 113
    cervical 55, (68) 97
    first (29) 57, (65) 95
right atrial appendage (83) 108
right colic artery 173
right portal vein (159) 176
roots of teeth (7) 44
rostrum, corpus callosum (18) 50
rotator cuff 137, (121) 139, (257) 271
rugae 174

sacralization, L5 vertebra (148) 169
sacroiliac joint (184) 202, (189) 205, (199) 210, (213) 233, (262) 274
sacrum (184) 202
    ala (212) 232, (251) 268
    canal (189) 205
    foramina (199) 210
    lumbo-sacral junction (148) 169, 170
    unfused joint (189) 205
sagittal suture (4) 42
sail sign 99
Santorini, duct of (166) 180, 181
saphenous nerve 271
sartorius muscle 237, (251) 268, (256) 271
scalene muscles (39) 62
scalenus anterior muscle 105, (90) 112–13, (92) 114
scapho-lunate joint (131) 144
scaphoid (130) 143, (132) 144, (134) 145
scapula (29) 57, (66) 95, (70) 99
    acromion process (116) 136, (121) 139
    coracoid process (70) 99, (117) 137, (120) 138
    spine (38) 61, (71) 99, (117) 137, (121) 139
sciatic nerve (217) 236
segmental pulmonary arteries (67) 96
segments
    bronchopulmonary 104–5, 109
    kidney 177
    liver (155) 173
semicircular canals (24) 54
semimembranosus muscle 237
seminal vesicle (198) 209, (200) 210, (264) 275
semitendinosus muscle 237
septa (cardiac)
    interatrial (82) 107
    interventricular (89) 112
septum pellucidum (18) 50, (250) 268

serratus anterior muscle (79) 104, 275
sesamoid bones
    of thumb (130) 143, 144
    plantar (230) 244
Shenton's line (212) 232
short saphenous vein 241
shoulder
    MRI (120) 138
    trans-scapular view (117) 137
sigmoid colon (153) 172
sigmoid sinus 47
silhouette sign 94
sino-atrial node artery (76) 102, 107
sino-tubular junction (83) 108
sinus venosus 267
sinuses of Valsalva 108
skull (1) 41
    base (8) 45
        lines (35) 60
    child (5) 43
    Towne's view (4) 43
small-bowel follow-through (151) 170–1
soft palate (18) 50, 51
soft tissues
    plain radiographs (184) 202, (251) 268
    prevertebral (27) 56
soleal line 269
soleus muscle 245, (252) 269
spermatic cord (194) 207, (217) 236
sphenoid bone, lesser wing (10) 46
sphenoid sinus (1) 41, (18) 50
sphincter of Oddi 181
sphincters
    anus (194) 207
    urethra (196) 208
spinal accessory nerve (90) 112
spinal cord (167) 181–2
    upper cervical (37) 61
spinal nerve roots
    brachial plexus 114
    cervical (39) 62, (260) 273, (263) 274
    ganglia (91) 113
    lumbar (262) 274
    sacral (199) 210, (246) 266, 274
spinous processes, vertebrae (66) 95
    C4 (26) 55
    C7 (27) 56
spleen (254) 270
splenic artery (152) 171
splenic vein (159) 176
splenium, corpus callosum (18) 50
splenius muscle (38) 61
splenorenal ligament (158) 175
stations, mediastinal lymph nodes 97
sternocleidomastoid muscle (34) 59, (37 & 38) 61, (39) 62,
    (92) 114, (260) 273
sternocostal joints (73) 100, 101
sternohyoid muscle 59, (260) 273
sternothyroid muscle 59, (260) 273
sternum (73) 100, 101, (92) 114
stomach (147) 168, 174
    fundus (71) 99, (78) 104, 174

pyloric antrum (151) 170, 174
straight sinus (11) 46–7
strap muscles 59, (260) 273
stripes, pleural reflections 98
stylohyoid ligaments 57
styloid process
    radius (130) 143
    ulna (131) 144, (259) 272
sub-carinal lymph nodes (68) 97
sub-phrenic space (258) 272
subacromial space (121) 139
subarachnoid cisterns
    ambient cistern (12) 47
    pontine cistern (13) 48
subarachnoid spaces, neonates (15) 49
subclavian artery (39) 62, (72) 100, (79) 104, 105, 107
    aberrant 103, (88) 111
subclavian vein (39) 62
subdural haemorrhage 49
subfertility 204
subsartorial canal (256) 271
subscapularis muscle (88) 111, (118) 137, (120) 138, (257)
    271
subscapularis tendon (93) 115
substantia nigra (22) 52, 53
subtalar joint (226) 242, (229) 244
superficial cerebral veins (15) 49
superficial circumflex iliac artery (214) 234
superficial femoral artery (214) 234, 271
superficial palmar arch (128) 142, (259) 272
superior colliculi 49, (20) 51, (22) 52, (20 & 21) 52
superior medullary velum (35) 60
superior mesenteric artery 171, (154) 172, (155) 173,
    272
superior mesenteric vein (155) 173
superior oblique muscle (eye) (23) 53
superior orbital fissure (2) 42
superior petrosal sinus 47
superior rectal artery (186) 203
superior sagittal sinus (11) 46–7, (15) 49
superior vena cava (64) 94
    double (249) 267
suprarenal gland (adrenal gland) (156) 174, (164) 179
suprarenal vein 179
supraspinatus muscle (38) 61, (121) 139, (257) 271
supraspinous ligament (1) 41
surgical neck, humerus (116) 136
suspensory ligament of ovary (192) 206
suspensory ligaments of Cooper (74) 101
sutures, skull 43
    see also named sutures
swallowing 61
swimmer's view (29) 57
sylvian fissure (13 & 14) 48, (17) 50
symphysis pubis (184) 202, (213) 233
synovial fluid, gleno-humeral joint (119) 138

taeniae coli (148) 168
talocalcaneal joint (226) 242
talocalcaneal ligament (229) 244
talofibular joint (229) 244
talotibial joint (228) 243

talus (226) 242
tarsal bones (231) 245, (255) 270
teeth (7) 44, (28) 56
    orthopantomogram (6) 44
temporal horns, lateral ventricles (16) 49
temporal lobe *see* anterior temporal lobe
temporalis muscle (36) 60
temporomandibular joint (254) 269
tennis elbow 141
tensor fascia lata muscle (218) 237, (251) 268
tentorium cerebelli (21) 52
teres major muscle (121) 139, (257) 271, (265) 275
teres minor muscle (121) 139, (257) 271
testicular artery (201) 211
    see also gonadal artery
testicular vein (258) 272
testis (193) 206-7
thalamus (19) 51
    massa intermedia (20) 51
thenar eminence 145, (135) 146
third ventricle (12) 47
thoracic duct (77) 103
thoracic spine (29) 57, (87) 110-11, (91) 113, (156) 174
three column principle, lumbar spine 170
thumb, sesamoid bones (130) 143, 144
thymus 95, (70) 99
thyrohyoid membrane 55
thyroid cartilage (26) 55, (33) 59
thyroid gland (34) 59
    blood supply 270
tibia (219) 238
    condyles (252) 269
    malleoli (255) 270
    paediatric (220) 238
    tuberosity (222) 239
tibial nerve 236
tibialis anterior muscle (228) 243, (231) 245
tibialis posterior muscle (225) 241, (227) 242-3, 245
tibiofemoral space 238
Tom, Dick and Harry (mnemonic) 243
Tom, Harry and Dick (mnemonic) 243
Towne's view, skull (4) 43
trachea (66) 95, (72) 100, (249) 267
tracheal rings (33) 59, (34) 59
tracheobronchial lymph nodes (68) 97
trans-scapular view, shoulder (117) 137
transverse colon (153) 172, (159) 176
transverse fissure (85) 109
transverse ligament, atlas (31) 58
transverse processes
    cervical vertebrae (30) 57
    lumbar vertebrae (148) 168
transverse venous sinus (4) 42
transversus abdominis muscle (162) 178
trapezium (132) 144, (133) 145
trapezius muscle (38) 61, 113, (93) 115, (257) 271
trapezoid (bone) (131) 144, (133) 145
trapezoid component, coracoclavicular ligament (116)
    136
triangular cartilage 143-4, (131) 144
tricuspid valve (89) 112
trigeminal nerve (25) 54-5

basal foramina and (8) 45
trigone parietale 96
triquetral (134) 145
triradiate cartilage, acetabulum (213) 233
trochlea (127) 142
true pelvic floor (urogenital diaphragm) 204, (196)
    208
tubercle of intercondylar eminence (219) 238
tunica vaginalis (193) 207
turbinates, inferior nasal (23) 53, (253) 269

ulna (126) 141, (129) 143, (132) 144
    coronoid process (126) 141, (247) 266
    styloid process (131) 144, (259) 272
ulnar artery (128) 142, (133) 145
ulnar collateral ligament (247) 266-7
ulnar nerve (133) 145, (257) 271
ulnar vein (124) 140, (133) 145
ultrasound
    common femoral vein 235
    female reproductive tract (190) 205, (191) 206
    ovary (192) 206
    portal veins 179
    testis (193) 206-7
umbilical artery (149) 169
umbilical vein (149) 169, (159) 176
uncinate process, pancreas 179
ureter 177, 203
urethra (188) 204, (195 & 196) 208
    prostatic (188) 204, (200) 210
urogenital diaphragm 204, (196) 208
uterus (190) 205
    MRI (197) 209
uvula (263) 274

vagina (187) 204, (190) 205, (196) 208
    fornices 209, (246) 266
vagus nerve (78) 104, (86) 110
valves (cardiac) (69) 98, (254) 270, (261) 273
    aortic (69) 98, (83) 108, (254) 270
    mitral (69) 98, (89) 112, (261) 273
    tricuspid (89) 112
valves, venous (124) 140
valvulae conniventes 171
vas deferens (193) 207
vastus lateralis muscle (218) 237
vastus medialis muscle (256) 271
veins 235, 267
    valves (124) 140
venous pumps 269
venous sinuses, skull (11) 46-7
    see also transverse venous sinus
ventral duct of Wirsung 181
ventral spinal nerve roots 273
ventricles (brain)
    lateral ventricles, temporal horns (16) 49
    third ventricle (12) 47
    see also fourth ventricle
ventricles (heart) (64) 94
    moderator band (89) 112
vermis (21) 52
vertebra prominens (27) 56

vertebrae
  cervical (26) 55, (30) 57
  laminae (87) 110, 170, (260) 273
  lumbar (150) 169–70
  presacral (148) 168
  thoracic (87) 110–11, (91) 113, (156) 174
  see also pedicles; spinous processes
vertebral artery (30) 57, (37) 61, (40) 62
vesico-ureteric junction (185) 203
vestibular nerve (24) 54
vocal cords 55, 59

Wirsung, duct of 181

wisdom teeth (7) 44
Wrisberg's ligament (223) 240
wrist (130) 143–4
  adolescents (259) 272

xiphisternal joint 101

Y-Y line (213) 233

zygoapophyseal joints (27) 56, (91) 113, (150) 169
zygoma, frontal process (8) 45
zygomatic arch (3) 42